Notes on Being A Man

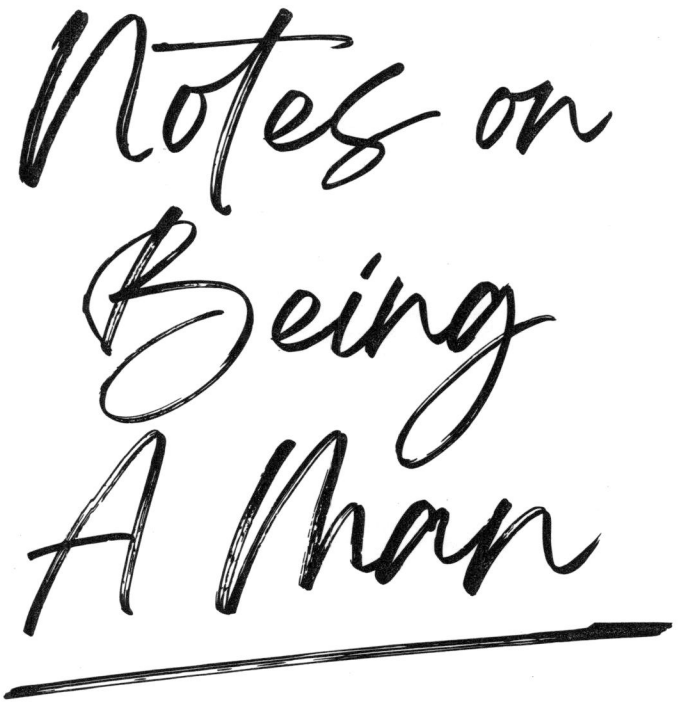

SCOTT GALLOWAY

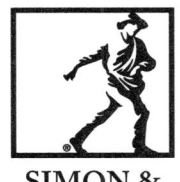

SIMON & SCHUSTER

London · New York · Amsterdam/Antwerp · Sydney/Melbourne · Toronto · New Delhi

First published in the United States by Simon & Schuster, an imprint of
Simon & Schuster LLC, 2025

First published in Great Britain by Simon & Schuster UK Ltd, 2025

Copyright © Scott Galloway, 2025

The right of Scott Galloway to be identified as the author of this work has been asserted in accordance
with the Copyright, Designs and Patents Act, 1988.

1 3 5 7 9 10 8 6 4 2

Simon & Schuster UK Ltd
1st Floor
222 Gray's Inn Road
London WC1X 8HB

For more than 100 years, Simon & Schuster has championed authors and the stories they create.
By respecting the copyright of an author's intellectual property, you enable Simon & Schuster and the
author to continue publishing exceptional books for years to come. We thank you for supporting
the author's copyright by purchasing an authorised edition of this book.

No amount of this book may be reproduced or stored in any format, nor may it be uploaded to any website,
database, language-learning model, or other repository, retrieval, or artificial intelligence system without express
permission. All rights reserved. Enquiries may be directed to Simon & Schuster, 222 Gray's Inn Road,
London WC1X 8HB or RightsMailbox@simonandschuster.co.uk

Simon & Schuster strongly believes in freedom of expression and stands against censorship in all its forms.
For more information, visit BooksBelong.com.

www.simonandschuster.co.uk
www.simonandschuster.com.au
www.simonandschuster.co.in

Simon & Schuster Australia, Sydney
Simon & Schuster India, New Delhi

The authorised representative in the EEA is Simon & Schuster Netherlands BV,
Herculesplein 96, 3584 AA Utrecht, Netherlands. info@simonandschuster.nl

Some names and identifying details have been changed.

The author and publishers have made all reasonable efforts to contact copyright-holders for permission, and
apologise for any omissions or errors in the form of credits given. Corrections may be made to future printings.

A CIP catalogue record for this book is available from the British Library

Hardback ISBN: 978-1-3985-5455-9
Trade Paperback ISBN: 978-1-3985-5456-6
eBook ISBN: 978-1-3985-5458-0

Interior design by Lewelin Polanco

Chart design by Olivia Reaney-Hall

Printed and Bound in the UK using 100% Renewable Electricity at CPI Group (UK) Ltd

Dedicated to:

George Thomas Galloway (Dad)
Terry Thomas (Mom's boyfriend)
Bernard Levene (uncle)
David Greene (uncle)
Alan Shepero (great-uncle)
Cy Cerro (stockbroker)
Charlie Evans (friend of family)
Jeff Baron (Camp Cottontail counselor)
Charles Knobler (Troop 42 scoutmaster)
Joe Sedia (baseball coach)
Don Olsen (high school guidance counselor)
Robert Tanowitz (Westwood Park coach)
Ray Goldstone (UCLA dean of students)
Peter Weiler (UCLA associate dean of students)
Carter Cordner (boss, Morgan Stanley)
David Aaker (professor, Berkeley Haas)
James Levine (literary agent)
David Wirtschafter (WME agent)
George Jarvis (friend's dad)
Paul Fine (friend's dad)
Hamid Moghadam (investor)
Tully Friedman (investor)
Warren Hellman (investor)
Paul Stephens (investor)
Pat Connolly (client)
Gord Shank (client)
Tyler Johnston (client)
Jeff Bewkes (investor)
Larry Bohn (investor)
Paul Sagan (investor)
Todd Benson (board member)
Peter Henry (dean, NYU Stern)
Howard Lester (client)
Raghu Sundaram (dean, NYU Stern)
Russ Winer (professor, NYU Stern)
William Berkeley (entrepreneur)
Dennis Chantland (board member)
Gary Magnus (client)
Robert May (investor)
Rich Lyons (chancellor, UC Berkeley)
Gary Futterman (fraternity pledge father)
F. D. Wilder (client)
David Fialkow (investor)

Contents

	Introduction	1
1	Boyhood	11
2	Things Get Hairy: Adolescence	36
3	Higher Education	60
4	Work	74
5	Health	115
6	Friendship	148
7	Sex, Love, Marriage	174
8	Fatherhood	204
9	Man . . . ners	238
10	Life Is So Rich	245
	Conclusion: A Letter to My Sons	261
	Acknowledgments	267
	Notes	269

Notes on Being A Man

INTRODUCTION

In 2007, late in life, I became a dad for the first time, looking on unsteadily as my son was born. I didn't fall in love immediately, though soon enough I did. Three years later, our second son was born. More unconditional love, shadowed a few years later by worry about what I was seeing and hearing online and off.

One of the semi-exciting perks of being an academic and "thought leader" is uncovering data, especially when it's both obvious and hidden. The alarming state of American boys and men overtook my attention. I track closely the emails I get. Most are from parents, particularly mothers, concerned about their sons, along these lines: "I have a daughter who lives in Chicago and works in PR and another daughter who's at Penn. My son lives in our basement, vapes, and plays video games." Moms, not dads, were leading the charge. Others were either ignoring the problem or didn't want to talk about it. Absent, too, was any sober, data-driven analysis. The gag-reflex cultural response seemed to be *Wow, men are worse than we think*, and that the issues they face are a function of their awfulness, and haven't we spent the past forty years correctly focused on the struggles of other, more deserving groups?

I connected to the topic on a personal level. I thought back on where I came from, my mom's irrational passion for my well-being, the generosity of California taxpayers who made it possible for an unremarkable kid with mediocre grades to attend college and business school, and all the obstacles, temptations, and traps that could have easily hampered my socialization—smartphones, online dating, porn, gambling, video games, remote work. I wondered why what was happening to boys and young men was in fact happening and how I could raise my sons in a world where they—and males of any age—thrive.

The data around boys and young men is overwhelming. Seldom in recent memory has there been a cohort that's fallen farther, faster. Why? First, boys face an educational system biased against them—with brains that mature later than girls', they almost immediately fall behind their female classmates. Many grow up without male role models, including teachers—fewer men teach K–12 than there are women working in STEM fields—with Black and Hispanic school instructors especially underrepresented.

Post–high school, the social contract that binds America—work hard, play by the rules, and you'll be better off than your parents were—has been severed. Seventy-year-old Americans today are, on average, 72 percent wealthier than they were forty years ago. People under the age of forty are 24 percent less wealthy. The deliberate transfer of wealth from the young to the old in the United States over the past century has led to unaffordable and indefensible costs for education and housing, and skyrocketing student debt, all of which directly affect young men. It's why twenty-five-year-olds today make less than their parents and grandparents did at the same age, while carrying debt loads unimaginable to earlier generations. Neither the minimum nor the median wage has kept pace with inflation or productivity gains, while housing costs have outpaced both. As the costs of college have soared beyond the reach of most families, many of the manufacturing jobs that didn't require a college degree and were often a ticket to the middle class for (mostly) men have been offshored. A prohibitive real estate market is a contributing factor to why 60 percent of young men between the ages of eighteen and twenty-four live with their parents and one in five still live with their parents at age thirty. Stuck and unable to afford greater economic opportunities in nearby cities, they find the same crush and collision of density, stimulation, humanity, creativity, eroticism, and conversation that urban areas offer on their phones instead. In Manhattan, a four-hundred-square-foot apartment costs $3,000 a month. In its stead is a seventeen-square-inch mobile studio apartment costing roughly $42 a month, served up by AT&T, T-Mobile, or Verizon.

Meanwhile, algorithmically generated content on social media contributes to—and profits from—young men's growing social isolation, boredom, and ignorance. With the deepest-pocketed firms on the planet trying to convince young men they can have a reasonable facsimile of life on a screen, many grow up without acquiring the skills to build social capital or create wealth. The percentage of young men aged twenty to twenty-four who are neither in school nor working has tripled since 1980. Workforce participation among men has fallen below 90 percent, caused by a lack of well-paying jobs, wage stagnation, disabilities, a mismatch of skills and/or training, and falling demand for jobs traditionally held by prime-age men.

This is deadly. From 2005 to 2019, roughly seventy thousand Americans died every year from deaths of despair—suicide, drug overdoses, alcohol poisoning—with a disproportionate number of those fatalities being unemployed white males without a college degree. Excluding deaths caused by the opioid epidemic, America's suicide and alcohol-related mortality rate for all races is higher than it's been in a century. It's also a mating crisis, as women traditionally mate horizontally and up socioeconomically, whereas men mate horizontally and down. Up until the mid–twentieth century, homogamy—marriages between men and women from similar educational backgrounds—was more common than not. Today, hypogamy, where women marry men who have less education than themselves, is on the rise. When the pool of horizontal-and-up young men shrinks, there are fewer mating opportunities, less family and household formation, and not as many babies. Here's a terrifying stat: 45 percent of men ages eighteen to twenty-five have never approached a woman in person. And without the guardrails of a relationship, young men behave as if they have . . . no guardrails.

Meanwhile, the whole subject of what it means to be a man has become radioactive, infected by dialogues that feel more like disdain (e.g., "toxic masculinity") than a conversation meant to address the issue (and here I'm not even including trans people or the many variations of gender that exist today). If men are struggling, the thinking goes, it's their fault.

> **Note:** *there's no such thing as "toxic masculinity"— that's the emperor of all oxymorons. There's cruelty, criminality, bullying, predation, and abuse of power. If you're guilty of any of these things, or conflate being male with coarseness and savagery, you're not masculine; you're* anti-masculine.

Most media portray men as idiots with decent hearts or show a man overcoming his inherent stupidity, racism, or biases to become a better person. The aspirational role models for men—Captain America, James Bond, LeBron James, etc.—aren't attainable for most of us. Rarely, either, in my experience do they include someone trying to be a good man/person and making a living and being there for his family.

Why are we so averse to identifying and celebrating what's good about men and masculinity, and why does it matter? Because we won't prosper if we convince boys and young men that they're victims, or that they don't have to be persistent and resilient, or that their perspective isn't valuable. If we do, we'll end up with a society of old people and zero economic growth. If we can't convince young men of the honor involved and the unique contributions inherent in expressing what makes them male, we'll lose them to niche, rabid online communities. Young men were instrumental in some of the most seminal events of the twentieth century, many if not all of which required collective effort, incredible bravery, risk-taking, aggression, and sacrifice. Can we acknowledge how extraordinarily important, skilled, strong, and decent most young men were carrying out the roles they played in helping create the world we live in? Some random examples include:

The Empire State Building was built by men. Construction began in 1930 and ended a year later, under budget and ahead of schedule. Among the 3,400 workers were carpenters, steelworkers, plumbers, bricklayers and derrick operators. Most made $15 a day. Two years later, *King Kong* made the roof famous.

Straddling Arizona and Nevada, the Hoover Dam generates hydroelectric power for three U.S. states. Construction took five years and gave birth to Lake Mead, which stores up to 9.2 trillion gallons of water. Around twenty thousand men showed up in Las Vegas a year after the start of the Great Depression to begin work in one-hundred-plus-degree weather. Sixteen workers died of heat prostration, countless others from carbon monoxide poisoning.

The soldiers who stormed the Normandy shores on D-Day, and who later fought and won the Battle of the Bulge, were young men. When Germans or Russians are streaming over the border or firing from the beach, big-dick energy isn't just a nice idea; it's fucking mandatory. The Battle of the Bulge was the final, deadliest offensive of World War II. Two hundred thousand German troops and one thousand tanks gathered in the Ardennes Forest in the winter of 1944—a last-ditch attempt on Germany's part to push the Allies back from home territory. The fighting went on for forty-one days, in subzero temps. It was awful. The Allies won, the American Army losing nineteen thousand men and suffering seventy-five thousand casualties.

I've often said history's greatest innovation isn't the semiconductor or the iPhone; it's the American middle class. It's not a naturally occurring organism—it'll go away unless income gets redistributed from upper income to middle income. The world works where a small number of very talented, well-connected, lucky people jump out ahead, use relationships and capital to pull farther away from the pack, and end up garnering a disproportionate amount of resources. Time passes, and the bottom 99 percent realize the quickest way to double their assets is to kill the top 1 percent. Then it starts all over again. It's the way of the world—a few extremely charmed (male) victors squeezing out all the other guys. It's why, historically and globally, many more females have passed on their DNA to their offspring than males.

Like most great and lasting inventions, the middle class was, in fact, a bit of historical freakery. At the center were seven million physically fit, nice-looking men who'd served in World War II, where they demonstrated masculine excellence; i.e., the ability to protect us from our enemies. They wore uniforms, were modest about their heroism, and were strong, and the United States, grateful and possibly starstruck, decided to give them money via the GI Bill, FHA loans, and the National Highway Transportation Act. A clean uniform, some money—and what do you know: women found these men attractive, and marriage, babies, and loving, secure households ensued. In sum, the greatest innovation in history grew out of an environment of attractive, heroic young men—Peak Male, if you will. It can happen again if we *make* it happen.

Female advancement in the past three decades is stunning. No one should want to slow the arrow of this trajectory. Overdue attention should be paid not just to girls and women but many other groups that history hasn't benefited the same way it has men. But empathy isn't a zero-sum game—it should be inclusive, not some *Hunger Games* competition for dwindling resources. Many people and groups today are suffering and in need of investment, attention, and support. But there's no escaping the fact that we see—and are continuing to create—a generation of young men from all backgrounds who are (a) unbearably lonely, (b) not economically viable, (c) not emotionally viable, and (d) basically adrift. And there is nothing more dangerous than a lonely, broke young man. It's a malevolent force in any society, and a truly terrifying one in a society addicted to social media and awash in guns and loutishness. Again, I connected to this topic on a personal level. *There but for the grace of God*, I thought—or would have if I thought such things.

I'm a faculty member at NYU's Stern School of Business. I teach a course called Brand Strategy, not The Issues Facing Boys and Men. I'm not an athlete, a politician, an ex-SEAL, or an evangelist. I have no training on the subject of boys and men, either as an academic or a therapist. I haven't devoted my life to being a good man, a good citizen—when I was younger, my sole focus was on becoming wealthy. Being rich makes you rich; it doesn't make you a better man. But having spent the past six decades in a male body while watching a parade of fake men selling distorted versions of what it means to be a man, I have some thoughts.

I grew up in Southern California in the late 1960s and early 1970s, an era marked by *The Partridge Family*, Sea-Monkeys, and Leo Sayer. I'm the only son of a single mom, whom I lost too soon in my thirties and whom I think about and miss every day. My dad left when I was nine or ten. Aside from a few sparks of early promise, I was an unremarkable boy, teen, college and B-school student. I was married and divorced by thirty-four. I've founded nine companies, several have been successful, and their success has led to a media business that is rewarding both economically and emotionally. I remarried, to a wonderful woman, and we have two teenage boys, all of whom I love deeply. I fly around the world giving speeches, taping podcasts, and making occasional TV appearances. I'm a loner, an introvert who's dealt his whole life with mild depression and anger issues. Again, you won't find my face on a poster over any young man's bed.

This didn't keep me from wondering: Why isn't anyone out there defending and championing men? The walls lining the NYU corridors are colorfully postered with announcements, meetings, and get-togethers for groups ranging from student bagpipers to Morris dancers. If there's anything specifically for men, it's assumed to be some shadowy cabal. This indifference extends to the Democratic National Committee, whose website has a page titled "Who We Serve." Listed are sixteen constituencies, including African Americans, the LGBTQ+ community, women, veterans and military families, and a dozen other demographic groups. Conspicuously missing are boys and men. Men have had twenty years experiencing what women and many groups have experienced for two thousand years—but wasn't the lesson to make room for everyone in the conversation?

Families feel this. I believe the 2024 election was about struggling young people, especially struggling young men. If your son is in the basement vaping and playing video games, you don't really care about trans athletes or territorial sovereignty in Ukraine; you just want change—that is, chaos and disruption. Seeing this, the Trump campaign flew into the manosphere with coarse language, crypto, Rogan, UFC, and Hulk Hogan. Donald Trump gained 16 percent with young men in 2024—the biggest pivot from Democrats to Republicans of any age group. Another big shift was among women aged forty-six to sixty-four, who, I believe, are the mothers of struggling young men. The election was supposed to be a referendum on women's rights. It was instead a referendum on failing young men.

Despite the significant age difference between my sons and me, I believe there are certain givens about what it means to be male. Most don't become dated or expire. I think of masculinity as a three-legged stool. Those legs provide a path forward for boys and men today. In answer to the questions *Why are men here?* and *What do men do?* the answer is threefold: Men Protect, Provide, and Procreate.

Protect: If you're looking for a good shorthand phrase for healthy masculinity in 2025, you could do a lot worse than the word "mensch," which in German simply means "human" and in Yiddish describes "a person of integrity or rectitude; a just, honest, or honorable person." The first instinct of a mensch is to protect, to sacrifice for something bigger than oneself, and not to pick on the vulnerable but to look out for your family and community. Real men don't start bar fights; they break them up. They don't shit-post other people or their country; they defend both. A man's default setting should be to move to protect, in any situation.

Provide: Historically, being a provider was a man's job. But women also becoming breadwinners doesn't mean the role is any less important for men. At the outset of his career, every man should assume he needs to take economic responsibility for his household. A man with a decent job in a strong economy is creating wealth, paying taxes, and earning social capital, not to mention his own self-respect. He also provides stability, support, love, and trust for his family, community, and himself. He's a ballast that absorbs the dramas taking place around him without giving in to them himself. Also, being a provider sometimes means getting out of the way of a wife or partner who may be better at the money thing and picking up the slack elsewhere—all the while being supportive.

Procreate: The third foundational element of masculinity is ensuring the species endures. This doesn't mean having children is an obligation—many people can't or choose not to and are instead great uncles, aunts, cousins, friends, and mentors—but arguably it's why we're here. This starts with . . . sex. My generation never gave up on sex. However, lately, underemployed and screen-numb young men, who feel rejected in an increasingly winner-take-all dating market, have thrown in the towel. Meanwhile, young women find themselves in an intensifying competition for a shrinking pool of what they view as viable mates. The viral hit is "I'm looking for a man in finance or media," not "I'm looking for a high school dropout who lives with his parents." Being a procreator doesn't mean having sex with as many women as possible or having no contact with your kids. A good procreator invests time, energy, and resources to raise kids who are stronger, smarter, faster, and more impressive than him.

The ultimate goal for any male is to create what the author of *Of Boys and Men*, Richard Reeves (my Yoda on this subject), calls *surplus value*. This phrase shows up a lot in these pages. It means you give more than you get. For men, this means providing more love to others than was given to you—becoming a better son, brother, friend, or employer to people. Your job, if you become a father, is to create surplus value as measured by being a better dad than your dad was to you.

Why does this topic preoccupy me? An easy answer is that my two boys have brought me more joy and satisfaction than anything else in my life. This book comes out of concern for their well-being and my desire, shared by all parents of sons, to see them lead productive lives. As my boys see me as uncool and lame, they won't read this book. I hope others do.

These pages are structured loosely as a memoir. They're organized chronologically on my journey from boyhood to manhood. (Note: I'm still learning.) The thoughts in here are observations, not peer-reviewed academic research or a road map sketched by someone who has arrived. Like most men, I'm a work in progress. I bring to the subject curiosity and no greater level of expertise than some research combined with my own biology, perceptions, and perspectives, including the times I've fucked up and been an egregious excuse for a man/human. I'm not saying what's in this book is the right way, but it's my way. I hope my story resonates and intersects with the lived experiences of other groups, as many of the issues outlined here are especially acute for nonwhite males. A decent percentage of the population will have a different view and outlook. I get that, and as a white, heterosexual male, I don't purport to have the skills or life experience to tell others what it means to be a man. I ask you instead to mull your own passage and relationship with masculinity: What's your own story? Ultimately, this book is about what it means from my perspective to be a responsible human flooded with testosterone and to encourage us to embrace an aspirational vision of masculinity that can serve as a code going forward.

As my *Pivot* podcast cohost Kara Swisher commented once, it should matter to everyone if men aren't thriving. Women and children can't flourish if men aren't doing well. Neither will our country.

chapter 1

BOYHOOD

"I DIDN'T SEE IT."

My best friend, since the fifth grade, is Adam Markman—for the past fifty years we've spoken nearly every week. Similar to mine, Adam's parents divorced when he was young. Unlike mine, Adam's mom returned to law school, where she met and married Paul, a handsome man ten years her junior. Paul looked like an Italian Kris Kristofferson, a quiet alpha male who possessed the key attribute of impressive men in seventies and eighties California: awesome cars. A Datsun 240Z, a Porsche 911, and then the pinnacle of Southern California manhood, a Ferrari. Their awesomeness was a footnote to his career progression as a lawyer defending insurance companies.

Paul and Adam's mom, Dvorah, have been together fifty years. She is struggling now with late-stage dementia and Paul, despite the urging of their kids, refuses to put her in assisted living and is essentially her full-time nurse. If I could encapsulate a feeling, a notion of what it is like to be a man, in a picture and show it to my sons, it might look like Paul. A handsome man, always working out, successful, a good father to his stepchildren, unflappable, and now a full-time caregiver, tending to his wife of fifty years. I've never heard anything remotely resembling a complaint from Paul. A few images come to mind: him (handsome); his kindness; his Ferrari; laughing at off-color jokes with friends over for *Monday Night Football*; and holding Dvorah's hand at lunch as she repeatedly called me Adam. Paul is a good man.

Growing up, Adam and I spent more time at his house than at mine for two reasons: the vibe at Adam's was more fun since he had an older sister (Jill) we could terrorize and Paul had other impressive men over to watch football; and his mom was a better cook. My mom's British roots and full-time job made for a cocktail of food as punishment. I still find eating a nuisance and have always struggled to keep weight on. But this story isn't about my body dysmorphia or Adam; it's about Paul.

Ten years ago, Paul was visiting New York, and I invited him to come by L2, the business intelligence firm I founded and later sold to Gartner.

L2, which took up two floors and had an open layout, defined a new generation of Gotham business. It was cool, intense, and alive, littered with impressive young people in conference rooms alongside less cool clients transfixed by roughly twelve hundred data points highlighting the strengths and weaknesses of their digital footprint relative to their peer group.

I felt proud and, despite his stoic demeanor, I could tell Paul was impressed. We took seats at a desk, where I walked him through what L2 did. An analyst stopped by to show visualizations of consumer engagement on Instagram—Estée Lauder versus L'Oréal. The in-house studio was the last stop, where another cohort of L2 employees was filming a video about e-commerce trends in China. It felt like a scene from *Mad Men*, if the show's final season were set in 2017 New York and Don Draper was dramatically less handsome.

As I walked Paul to the elevator, I felt his hand on my shoulder. "Scott, I have to be honest." He paused, turned, and looked at the expanse of the office, then returned his gaze to me. "I didn't see it."

I found this strangely rewarding. It was honest, and true. There was nothing in my upbringing or how I acquitted myself that would have predicted success. A few years ago, I went to my thirtieth high school reunion. By then I'd achieved some level of celebrity/notoriety. Few classmates remembered me. If they had, I would have thought there was something wrong with them. The past is prologue to everything and nothing. A big part of my belief system—where I give money and the issues I focus on—is shaped by a belief that no person or institution can predict greatness or failure in an eighteen-year-old, much less an eight-year-old. America is about watering as many plants as possible, not attempting to determine which seeds will become redwoods.

ORIGIN STORY

Everyone has an origin story: we define ourselves by our backgrounds—what and who made us who we are. But we often don't let the truth get in the way of a good story. The narrative of "I" is often just that: a story. It can sound like a high-concept elevator pitch. The more honest, nuanced version of who we are belongs to our friends, our partners, and our therapists (if we have them). This is mine: how family, circumstances, timing, culture, women, and other boys and men helped me get where I am.

In the second grade, I was the only son in a nuclear family where Dad was a vice president for International Telephone & Telegraph (ITT) and Mom was a secretary. We lived in a house overlooking the Pacific in Laguna Niguel. That's in Orange County. My parents were both living the American Dream. Two immigrants, my mom English, my dad Scottish, both with eighth-grade educations, they raised sails, hard work, and talent to the greatest gale force wind in history: the U.S. economy. We lived near enough to the beach that if you stood on your toes in the living room, you could see a narrow ribbon of blue. Our home had an "ocean view."

Dad: one of my strongest, and first, memories was noticing how people behaved around him. As early as five, I saw they treated him differently than everyone else. They would fix on his eyes, nodding and then laughing. Women would touch his arm, giggling, and men, when they saw him, would yell "Tommy!" and be genuinely happy to see him. My dad was great with a turn of phrase, and clever (i.e., Scottish). The cocktail of articulate, irreverent, and smart chased with a Scottish accent made him attractive to women and employers. Especially women. My mom was his second wife; two more were on deck.

My mother's explanation when I queried her about this effect he had on people: "Your father is charming." This charm sustained, for a decade, an upper-middle-class lifestyle for him, my mom, and me as he roamed the Western United States and Canada, fostering, in fifteen-minute spurts, pseudofriendships with managers of the outdoor and garden departments at Sears and Lowe's. In exchange for his company, my dad's two hundred friends would over-order bags of shit . . . as he was selling fertilizer from O.M. Scott, an ITT company.

Mom: growing up, my dad liked to remind me that a twenty-one-mile strip of water, the English Channel, saved my life. My mom—I talk about her a lot; she would have liked that—was four, a Jew, and living in London when World War II broke out. Before she was moved to the British countryside, along with the other kids in Central London, she and her family would sleep in the tube—the subway, which had become a makeshift bomb shelter, where the adults passed out gas masks. The kids' masks had rubber duck-like bills and funny ears to make them, and what was happening, less scary.

Both my parents took huge risks coming to America. Why? Because they wanted to work their asses off and be rewarded for the risks they were willing to take. This is capitalism, a promise of prosperity for people who are smart, hardworking, and comfortable with risk, promising a greater share of the spoils than to those who are not. Living in London and doing fifty-plus speaking gigs a year, when speaking to UK audiences I'm often asked to compare and contrast the U.S. and the UK. "In sum," I like to say, "America is an organism whose DNA was inherited from people who all took risks"—pause—"and you're the ones who stayed."

At the same time, so much of success and failure is random and accidental. A good percentage comes down to when and where you were born.

My mom, Sylvia, had a great sense of humor. She loved to laugh and was always a hard worker, a good friend, and a kind, loving person. There was never any doubt I was the most important thing in her life. I miss her a great deal.

Me: so much I didn't know. For example, I didn't appreciate that being born when and where I was meant I'd already won the lottery. I was a mediocre kid with the good fortune to be a white, heterosexual male born in sixties California, meaning some of the finest educational institutions in the world would let me attend for free.

Before my parents divorced, my dad would come home early from work and we'd go bodysurfing and see seals and porpoises just offshore. When there was a storm, in the morning we'd go to Newport Beach. From the end of the pier, we'd look several hundred feet out and alert each other when millions of gallons, barreling toward shore, morphed into a blue-gray hemicylinder, eight, maybe ten feet high, and wait for the pier to shake as the rising seafloor thrust the cylinder up and the wave crashed down on the water. One of four consecutive nights, beginning on the full and new moons in spring, my mom would wake me at midnight and, armed with flashlights, we'd traipse down to the beach and watch what looked like hot slices of metal dancing in the shallow surf. The grunion—tiny, silvery fish that lay their eggs on the sand—were running.

TEED OFF

Did I know I was a boy or that gender would play a role in my opportunity set? No. The patriarchal handbook says boys and men are so used to being in the driver's seat, gunning the engine and flicking the lights, they forget they're driving.

The fix was in, though. How and in what ways I came to be born male was a fourfold process, as it is for all boys. A short detour into boyhood and male science:

Testosterone, or T, is an androgen. *Andro* is Latin for "man," and *gen* short for "generating." An androgen is any hormone that supports and promotes the development of male sex characteristics, the goal being to get young males reproducing. T is an incredible substance. It's the engine of masculinity, what wins wars and World Series. It plays a big role in fetal development in both sexes, though boys and men have anywhere from ten to twenty times as much as girls and women. Every embryo begins life as a female. The combo of the Y chromosome and testosterone causes male development in body and brain to diverge sharply from females.

The first flush of T happens in the womb. Along with determining male physiology and anatomy, T also increases male height relative to women. The role testosterone plays in creating a "male brain" is a subject that can lead to shouting matches in faculty lounges. Does T hijack boys' brains, compelling an interest in sharks, dinosaurs, trains, construction equipment, and weaponry, or are brains more like whiteboards that fall prey to culturally imposed blue and pink color schemes? My experience, mostly through the inexact science of observing my kids' playdates, is that, as Michelle Obama said, "They come to you." That is, it's more nature than nurture.

The scientific view is that T "masculinizes" the brain. Many take issue with this, as genetics, hormones, and the environment all come together to affect the development of anyone's brain. Everyone is born with the genetic equipment to express the spectrum of stereotypically "male" and "female" behavior, though the ratios differ. Some of the most wonderfully masculine people I know are women, and some of the best men I know demonstrate feminine attributes. A friend of mine is a hedge fund manager with a house in Montauk. Whenever I

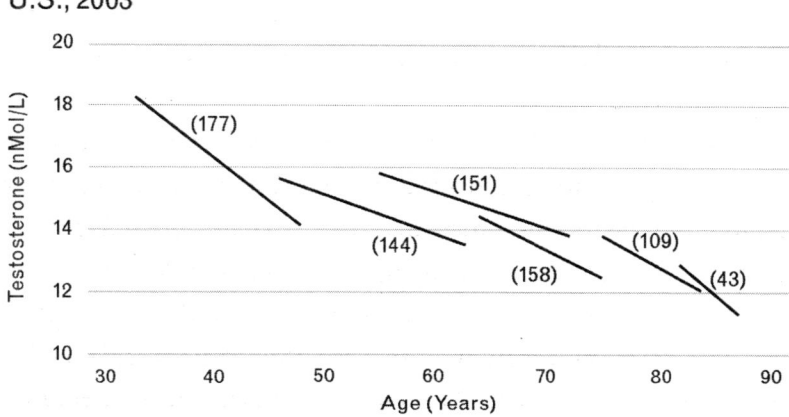

Source: Institute of Medicine of the National Academies, 2003. *Clinical Research Directions*: Testosterone and Aging.

visit, before I arrive, he turns down the sheets and lights a candle. He takes care of me.

If the first flush of T happens in utero, the second appears right after birth. The third shows up at the onset of puberty, when T inspires the male growth spurt, generating facial and body hair, sperm production, stronger, longer bones and increased muscle mass, and a deeper voice. T peaks at age twenty—the curtain call for puberty. From then on, like air slowly leaking from a tire, T declines. After the age of forty, T decreases roughly 1.2 percent a year. No man needs to be reminded of this. A few years ago, I started injecting testosterone. T makes me feel stronger, younger, and (supposedly) is brain- and heart-protective. Those aren't trivial benefits.

From a young age, T gives boys an innate athletic advantage over girls. Across cultures, boys roughhouse, hit each other, break windows, and turn expensive things into less valuable things. Some women find this perplexing—it's just T. When T goes up, so do motivation and reward, while fear and pain perception go down.

Ultimately, T has one role: to mix and merge male anatomy,

physiology, and behavior so that men gain access to a pool of potential mates and enhance their reproductive success. Translation: T's blind mission is to ensure the species continues via sex. Traits such as dominance, ambition, competition, confidence, skill, risk-taking, size, or anything that can help a man beat back competitors and attract a mate's attention are welcome. Yes, T can make boys and men reckless, stupid, and mean, but also valiant, fearless, and heroic.

GIFTED, FOR A WHILE

In the late 1950s, the Space Race went from a walk to a sprint. The Russians launched Sputnik, the world's first artificial satellite, into orbit. It was purposefully non-stealth, emitting radio signals across two frequencies. The steady beep, beep was an incessant reminder "they" were winning. The United States got to work, and elementary and middle school teachers were charged with identifying and matriculating a new generation of warriors. But these warriors were meant to be more Doogie Howser than Maximus Decimus Meridius (Russell Crowe's character in *Gladiator*). The key was to identify (mostly) boys whose genius could ultimately be weaponized against the Russkies.

Some people peak later in life—Julia Child, Colonel Sanders, Ray Kroc (something about food)—and others earlier on. Similar to a child movie star, I peaked at age eight. Debbie Brubaker and I were the smartest kids in Emelita Street Elementary School's third grade, as indicated by our math and English scores. Oddly, we were also the fastest girl/boy. One day, our teacher (Mrs. Marsh) called us to her desk and informed us we would be spending the mornings with the fifth-grade class.

I remember telling my mom, and she was so proud. Think about how much things have changed, and how trust in institutions has eroded; nobody from my school asked or even told my mom that I'd no longer be learning alongside kids my age. At the time, the third graders were learning the now-dead art of cursive. When Debbie and I got the news, we were scribing the letter "L" over and over in our notepads. To this day I can barely handwrite the letters between "M" and "Z."

Along with taking fifth-grade English and math, in fourth grade I was named to the San Fernando Valley all-star baseball team (pitcher and second base). I was also showing dim flashes of entrepreneurship, or possibly greed. At age nine, I had a paper route, walked three dogs, and sold magazine subscriptions door-to-door. In seventh grade, I would buy a pack of Bubble Yum for 15 cents at the local convenience store with five pieces to a pack. I resold them to my classmates for a nickel apiece. I'd chew half my profits, but still made money.

My friend Adam also had an aunt who coordinated product sponsorships for television game shows with brands including Rice-A-Roni and Turtle Wax. Thanks to her, we were beta-testers for a high-pressure hose that sprayed wax. Adam and I roamed Westwood, knocking on doors, offering a "wash and a wax for the price of a wash." I remember several customers negotiating us down from $4 to $3 when it rained, only to give us an extra $5 tip. Having odd jobs in Los Angeles instilled in me that, at their core, Americans are a generous people. I've tried to maintain this tradition.

My childhood golden years were meaningful but short lived. Soon, things started going downhill. I assumed I'd work in something to do with space, or science, while pitching for the California Angels. I'd be able to take care of my mom, show the Russians who was boss, while throwing no-hitters. Not in the cards.

SPLIT ENDS

When I was nine, my parents divorced. We were living the American Dream on the outside: two immigrants with a nice home and a thriving American son. However, the core was rotting. At that age, I could sense it . . . but not identify it. Whatever is going on in a nine-year-old's life has some sense of normalcy as you have so little to benchmark it against. Your situation, no matter how strange, is the standard. There was some foreshadowing: my parents were thickly silent at the dinner table, my mom so morose. A few times, I'd come downstairs in the morning to find my dad screaming at my mom. It usually had something to do with money she had spent on an object he felt was wasteful. She'd be sitting in a chair at our kitchen table in just her underwear, shivering and sobbing. He'd motion with his hand as if he was going to strike her, she'd recoil, and he'd circle the kitchen table, pick up a magazine or item from the shelf under our wall-mounted phone, and hurl it at her. When he was this angry, his Glaswegian accent would become near indecipherable. My dad would scream at me, and I'd retreat to the top of the stairs.

This is the part of the book where, if I were on the cusp of announcing my candidacy for public office, I'd lay out in cinematic detail how I stood up to my father. I didn't. Truth is I didn't know what the fuck to do. I'd sit at the top of the stairs, listening to this scene play out, over and over. Though it never became familiar.

> **Note:** *Being a good dad means being good to the mother of your children.*

Soon after and almost worse, ambivalence infected our home. Basically, my dad was no longer interested in my mom or me. He was spending time in Texas, engaged in a budding relationship with a woman who later became his third wife. It's tempting to depict her as a bad person. She isn't. In fact, she, Linda, was wonderful to me. During this time, my mom became either depressed or so fed up with my dad that she became indifferent, too, ignoring us both. It was an ocean-view home filled with . . . nothing. It wasn't what happened that made it such a depressing environment, but what didn't happen: absence versus presence. There was no affection, no teasing, no arguing, no discipline, no conversation. Nothing. The few times I think

I've been clinically depressed I didn't feel sad, I felt nothing. As if my feet were hollow and my being had experienced a brownout.

And then my mom disappeared for a few weeks. My dad said she was vacationing with friends. I remember asking what a vacation was, as I don't think we'd ever taken one as a family. My dad used to go on trips all the time, but not with us. As a salesman, then executive, for ITT, he was constantly going to Hilton Head or Phoenix with other salesmen to play golf, drink, and hear about a new incentive plan to motivate them to sell more (literal) shit.

One of his favorite stories is about me watching him, the evening before a trip, lay out his stuff—cashmere sweaters, pleated pants, his golf bag—and I asked my mom, "Why is Dad so rich and we're so poor?" He thought that was hilarious.

After she'd been gone for three weeks, my father announced he was going to the office and my mom would be back later that afternoon. My mom walked through the door and, before saying hello, told me to pack my stuff as we were leaving. "Where are we going?" I asked. Her only response, repeatedly, was "We're leaving." I remembered there had been talk of us getting a dog earlier, and, as nine-year-olds do, I thought this was an opportunity to bring up adding to the family. "Will we be able to get a dog?" "No." The whole situation, and its weirdness, became too much to handle and I put my arms around her waist and began sobbing. My mom was still for a second and then began vibrating and then convulsing. She was crying so hard.

Since then, I've had trouble dealing with women in pain. Not in a chivalrous way, but I have trouble functioning around women crying or in distress in any kind of way (i.e., I'm useless). When you're a kid, and your mom is your whole life, naturally you're going to worry about her. It's evolution: without your mom sheltering you and growling, you'll get eaten. For several years, when my mom appeared to be in pain—getting her ears pierced, frustrated with the broken vacuum—I'd feel sick. Several times, I passed out. Whether it's my mom, my wife, or any woman I'm close to, I just can't handle it. I get anxious and queasy, literally feeling like I'm about to collapse. It's embarrassing. Mostly it comes from the fear that I have no control, that I can't *do* anything.

Once my mom stopped shaking, I put all my clothes in grocery bags since we didn't own a suitcase, I loaded them in the back of her red Mercury Capri, and we left. The truth about her disappearance came out later. My mom had been hiding out with her friends Karsen and Charly after my dad said "I want custody of Scott" (California didn't implement joint custody laws until 1980). Leaving me alone with my dad was a ploy, a way of reminding my dad that he had zero aptitude, skills, resources, bandwidth, or inclination to parent a nine-year-old boy solo (he hadn't aced it thus far, married). Forty-eight hours into my stay, having sequestered me in a back room with a TV set and a TV dinner, my dad, neck misted lightly with Brut cologne, was already entertaining a sultry, dark-haired, presumably married female neighbor over two cold bottles of Lancers rosé. It took him less than a week to call my mom and say, "You can come get Scott."

My mom told me this last part during a car ride. Her exact words: "I knew your dad wouldn't want you after having you alone for three weeks." She didn't say it to be hurtful, and I don't remember being that upset about it. I absorbed it, is all. Today, I think, *Wow, forty-eight hours later, my dad was already hitting on other women.*

It was a different era. California in the 1970s was all about grown men and women awakening to submerged needs. The culture was one of self-absorption dressed in a mutable spirituality. Children were collateral damage, held hostage to parental stirrings. These days, every decision parents make is the tail (your kids) wagging the dog, every decision a function of what's best for them (your kids). "Birdnesting" is a trend today, where children stay in familiar bedrooms while their divorcing parents take turns squatting in the family home. This is meant to avoid disruption, at least for the child, though it sounds like hell for the parents. In the early 1970s, birdnesting would have been fodder for sci-fi books.

Within three months my parents were divorced. There was no

custody fight. Within six months, my dad moved to Ohio for a bigger, better job. From that point on, it was my mom and me against the world.

That world became measurably smaller. We moved from Laguna Niguel to an apartment in Tarzana, which was more inland and suburban. We went from living an upper-middle-class life to a lower-middle-class one in just one TV season. Same American Dream, this time in reverse. I changed schools. Either my brain slowed down or I was more affected than I thought by the divorce; things started going off the tracks for me. I went from being a precocious student and good baseball player to neither. My slow descent into unremarkableness was underway.

Most boys come apart when a male role model leaves. I went from seeing my dad every day to seeing him maybe every other month, along with summers and Christmas. Post-divorce, my mom and dad were the characters in a new series titled *Primitive Family*, in that they hated each other and made everything worse than it had to be. And it was the least funny thing in all our lives.

The divorce left my mom feeling angry, upset, economically strained, and traumatized. I'd wait outside, sometimes for an hour, a good distance from our apartment as my mom didn't want to risk seeing my dad, or even his car—she hated him that much. Occasionally, Dad's #3 (Linda) would call my mom to discuss logistics. Inevitably, after something pissed her off, my mom would slam down the phone, pause, look at me, and say, "I hung up on that bitch!"

I was angry on her behalf and would get angrier over time, but, like a premium brand, my dad's newfound scarcity made him an alluring figure. I'd gotten good at identifying cars from far off, by the shape and luminosity of their headlights. AMC Pacers were easiest. Alone on the sidewalk outside my mom's eight-hundred-square-foot apartment, I could spot my dad's Gran Torino in the dark from half a mile away. I was like a miniature ship in the waves, scanning the horizon for a light beam.

When I wasn't getting picked up or dropped off, I served as a go-between. "We need a TV," my mom would say. "Ask your dad." "I can't," I said, "it's too embarrassing." We both knew that my dad, raised in Depression-era Scotland, had a fucked-up relationship with money—especially when it came to other people (us) spending it. Whether it was ordering a shake at Baskin-Robbins, buying clothes, or discussing a vacation, spending money was verboten. Pre-divorce, our household wasn't economically anxious but stressed. My mom and I were always on edge, fearful we'd committed a crime against humanity anytime we spent money. Now it was worse.

In some fucked-up expression of independence, my mom didn't fight for alimony and instead received just $200 every month for child support. One month the check didn't arrive. As the indirect recipient of my dad's largesse, I was given verbal instructions for that weekend's visit. I was to tell my dad that if the check didn't show up, my mom would call his boss and tell him my dad was a deadbeat. I spent that entire weekend feeling incredibly nauseated. Finally, on the way back to my mom's, I delivered the message. "Tell your mom I'm not sending it," my dad said.

Hindsight is unfair and clarifying. My dad could have made our lives much easier. He could have eliminated a lot of our stress. It wouldn't have been that hard or costly, and he could have afforded it. But he didn't, and I came to resent him for it, and for how callous he was to my mom. This grated on me more than his lack of interest in me. Yes, he had many good qualities. He was—still is—charming, handsome, funny, a great storyteller. A Scottish accent and a robust jawline was the 1970s equivalent of today being in the top 10 percent of online dating. Living in 1970s California, my dad had a disproportionate number of mating opportunities. He could not only think with his dick but listen to it. People believe fidelity is correlated to morality. Maybe. My experience is it's inversely correlated to opportunity. Anybody marrying an athlete, actor, billionaire—someone who gets most, if not all, their self-esteem from their looks or has a Scottish accent—should assume that person will have sex with other people. My dad has been married and divorced four times—I have a half sister, Asheley, from marriage number three to Linda. He divorced his last wife (Marcia), of thirty-five years, three years after her Parkinson's diagnosis and two years before she passed away.

Pulled out of school in Scotland at thirteen to work as a messenger for maybe three shillings a week, he was unsophisticated. Both my parents were. He was also ambitious, though most of his confidence was sourced from women. Having grown up destitute, he was deathly afraid of being poor himself, which left us poorer and would later ignite the same feelings in me.

> **Note:** *Most boys come apart when a male role model leaves. If there is no father present, the son is more likely to be incarcerated than graduate from college.*

CADDYSHACKING

Ironically, after the divorce, my relationship with my dad improved in some ways. Presence-wise, of course, it suffered. He was no longer living with us, and so much of fathering comes down to sheer presence, i.e., being there. His marriage to his third wife helped. An exceedingly nice woman, Linda was blessed with parenting instincts my dad mostly lacked. A nice way of saying she would force him to spend time with me. "You're going golfing?" she would ask. "Then you're taking Scott with you." Off we went. It didn't matter that I had zero interest in golf. I'd walk around the course with him for four hours and try to spot his ball. I wouldn't even play—that would cost $8. That was okay, though, as I just wanted to be with him.

Some of our best times, in fact, involved golf, a game I gave up twenty years ago to free up more time for exercise. My dad and I would sneak onto some of Ohio's most exclusive golf courses at dusk with a 5 iron and a putter ("the only clubs you need"). My dad, like a skilled hunter, would find a clump of bushes that were sure to be teeming with golf balls given up by the rich and uncoordinated. Golf balls cost 11 cents to manufacture but retailed at $1.50 a sphere.

Like a fearless bird dog, I would dive into the foliage using my 5 iron as a makeshift machete. I wouldn't return until I saw a snake or procured six or more balls. We'd lay out our loot on the grass—a new Pinnacle! He'd point at it, nod, and then mess up my hair—his primary vehicle for affection. He did it often, and it felt wonderful. We'd then play six or seven holes with two clubs, never reserving or paying for tee time.

Our criminality graduated to seeing several movies on one admission ticket and (rarely, but more than once) dining and ditching. I wasn't a party to the latter. He'd pick me up from my mom's and we'd stop at Ships Coffee Shop in Westwood. After the meal, as his Gran Torino would accelerate from the Wilshire Boulevard artery feeding the 405, he'd look over and ask, "Did you pay?" I'd stare at him befuddled, and he'd say, "You're a wee scunner!" and laugh. Again, the mess of the hair, and it all seemed natural, wholesome even.

A couple of times, a course ranger in a golf cart emblazoned with badging that said (wait for it) RANGER or an exasperated waitress waving a check ran after us. As if wiping sweat from his brow, my dad would greet them with the welcome surprise of running into an old friend. He'd then break into the thickest Scottish accent; I mean, can't understand a word. He'd point at me a few times, pause, laugh, and put his hand on their shoulder. By this time they had bonded over the misunderstanding. My seventies Braveheart father would wink at me, and we'd leave the course or pay the check.

I'm convinced that the police could find my dad on top of a warm corpse with his hands wrapped around its throat, and he'd deploy his Lallans charm to get a ride home from the officers. Nothing can get you into trouble with women who aren't your wife, or out of trouble with service workers, better than a great jawline and a Glasgow twang.

Also, to his credit, my dad's parenting skills improved as he got older. He was a tangibly better dad to my half sister and even paid for her to go to grad school at Kellogg School of Management at Northwestern University. For my father, this was on par with the Marshall Plan.

But it was difficult to embrace someone when the most important person in my life, my mom, viewed him as her enemy. I couldn't help but see my dad through her lens, and that image was cloudy and aggrieved. Like many kids of divorce, I inflated the goodness of one parent at the expense of the other. My dad was on the wrong end of this stick. As a teenager, I resented my dad, as post-divorce his life—and his new family's—got better, and mine and my mom's got worse. Some of this was both of their doing, and some out of their control.

> **Note:** *Parents who infect their kids with their own trauma are super-spreaders. Divorced parents who infect their kids with their anger at their exes make both parents look bad.*

TETHERED

When I look at my own success, it mostly boils down to two factors: being born in America and having someone irrationally passionate about my well-being: my mom. Though she was raised in a household where there was little affection, my mom couldn't control herself with her son. For me, affection was the difference between *hoping* someone thought I was wonderful and worthy and *knowing* someone did.

Every Wednesday night after Boy Scouts, my mom and I would go to dinner at Junior's Deli. I would have the brisket dip, she the lox, eggs, and onions. We talked about our week—we didn't see each other much between weekends—only to be interrupted by different waitresses who would comment on how much I had grown. On the way out, we'd stop at the bakery and buy a quarter pound of halvah. As we stood in the parking lot waiting for the valet to retrieve our lime-green Opel Manta, my mom would grab my hand and, in an exaggerated fashion, swing it back and forth. She'd look at me, and I would return her gaze with an eye roll, at which point she would burst into joyous, uncontrollable laughter. She loved me so much.

Having a good person express how wonderful you are hundreds of times changes everything. College, professional success, an impressive mate—these were aspirations, not givens, for a remarkably unremarkable kid living in a household at the high end of the lower middle class. My mom was forty-three, single, and making $15,000 a year as a secretary. She was also a good person who made me feel connected and, while waiting for our Opel, gave me the confidence that I had value, that I was capable and deserving of more. Holding hands and laughing, I was tethered.

LONE SOLDIER PARENTING

In 1970s California, divorced kids not yet being a topic of conversation meant vigilant parenting wasn't, either. In its place was a cocktail of hope, trust, and fatalism.

My mom had little to no idea what I was up to most days. As a member of Gen X, I'd leave home Saturday morning with my Bahne skateboard, 35 cents, and an Abba-Zaba bar, not to be seen or heard from for twelve-plus hours. When I visited my dad in Ohio, she would drive me to the airport, we'd check in, and I'd get a small lapel sticker proclaiming I was a minor (either that or Paddington Bear). An airline representative was supposed to meet me at the gate. Sometimes they did, sometimes not.

At the age of eleven, the principal of Fairburn Elementary School knocked on our door and informed me, in my pajamas, that I needed to come back to school. My two-week self-imposed break from the sixth grade, binge-watching cartoons, had come to an abrupt end. I knew he could rat me out to my mom, who had no idea as she left each morning before me, so I agreed. He understood an unwritten code and never told her. I skipped the sixth grade for two weeks and my mom didn't notice (see above: a different era). Sort of a *Home Alone* times ten scenario with a single mom and a much less likable kid.

It wasn't like we had options. My mom and I weren't destitute, but money was always a thing. She raised me on her own, on a secretary's salary. Every day, she'd wake up at 6:30 so she could be in the car by 7:30 to make the drive over the hill into the Valley, where she oversaw the secretarial pool at an insurance firm and then downtown at the Southwestern School of Law. I remember getting sick at school, the nurse's office calling to say, "You need to come get Scott," and my mom saying, "I can't." She wasn't allowed to leave work. It would have meant an unpaid day off, or she might risk getting fired, sick kid or not.

Some givens fell naturally by the wayside. My first visit to the dentist, I had eight cavities. This was puzzling, given how little food I ate. My mom used to give me 55 cents for lunch, and I would pocket it and skip lunch. I used to have fainting spells, which prompted one of the first times I ever saw a doctor. He reeled off a series of questions, one being "What did you have for breakfast this morning?" "I didn't have breakfast," I said. "When's the last time you ate?" "I had cereal yesterday morning." My mom looked horrified, clearly concerned Child Protective Services was on the way. I just didn't eat a lot (still don't).

JEANNIE, GET BACK IN YOUR BOTTLE

My favorite shows as a kid were *The Brady Bunch* and *The Partridge Family*. These days, whenever I'm accused of saying anything sexist, my response is "Don't you realize how far I've come?" From the ages of eight to eleven, I was hooked on *I Dream of Jeannie*. Jeannie was a sexy two-thousand-year-old genie played by Barbara Eden, who lived inside a brass bottle and served as an enthusiastic slave and roommate to Larry Hagman, playing an astronaut named Tony Nelson. "Yes, Master, whatever you say," Jeannie would simper, to which Tony, exasperated, might snap, "Oh, Jeannie, get back in your bottle." *I Dream of Jeannie* was on four times a day.

A beautiful, eager-to-please woman in a low-cut top who lived inside a bottle—this was the cultural amniotic fluid I grew up in. The men on TV were mostly bumblers and morons. Among the exceptions were the Fonz from *Happy Days* and Steve Austin from *The Six Million Dollar Man*—the former a greaser, the latter a handsome, intelligent, athletic former astronaut whose body had been reconstructed from bionic machine parts, giving him gorilla strength, cheetah speed, and the admiration of a generation of teenage boys.

I also watched every one of the 168 episodes of *The Mary Tyler Moore Show*—with my mom, who, as a single working woman, identified with "Mary" (what my mom and her friends called her). The show broke new ground with episodes discussing infidelity, divorce, homosexuality, and addiction. However, the biggest breakthrough was portraying Mary Richards, a single woman on the wrong side of thirty as an independent, shit-together protagonist.

Throughout my working life, I've had formidable female cofounders and senior partners in all my companies. Nearly 80 percent of my senior management has been women or gay men. At first, I thought maybe I was threatened by straight men. But, no, my relationships with male clients and colleagues and employees were solid. Again, credit Mary Richards. She reminded me of my mom—a single woman trying to make it in the world who was more talented than anyone else in that newsroom. From early on, I remember thinking the most egregiously untapped professional resource was women, especially the ones I worked with. I offered them remote work before it was cool. It wasn't an effort to better the world; I've just always been comfortable around women and knew I could tap into great human potential with what felt highly unorthodox in the nineties: remote work.

Media's value is joy. Its value-add is fostering empathy. *The Mary*

Tyler Moore Show taught us that—even if a woman wasn't married with kids—friends, humor, and achievement could mean love was (still) all around.

ENEMIES OF YOUNG MEN: THE PREFRONTAL CORTEX

Growing up, I was drawn to novel, crazy experiences—in other words attracted to doing a wide variety of insanely stupid shit. So were most of my (male) friends. At age eight or nine, we would build ramps and jump with our bikes over one another's motionless bodies. I would skateboard down Wilshire Boulevard, not on the elbow or the sidewalk, but on the actual boulevard. The third and fourth grades of our school looked like an ER waiting room—casts, bandages, crutches, eye patches.

Then I got older, my incredible maturity obvious to everyone. In high school, I distinctly remember deciding *not* to study for the upcoming SATs—too boring and time-consuming. That same year, my mom had to sign a release so I could play on the high school baseball team, but I forgot to give it to her, which meant I wasn't allowed to play the first game and was eventually cut from the squad.

At UCLA, after my freshman year, I applied immediately for financial aid for the next year. I got a shit-ton, too, including Pell Grants. Then, a year later, aware that my junior year was coming up, I decided not to apply for financial aid, and, you know, whatever, take my chances.

Incredibly fucking stupid.

Other highlights from that era include never checking my car's oil level until the dashboard screamed with yellow and red symbols alerting me that either the engine was about to explode or a comet had just collided with Earth. When this car was later towed to a city pound—encumbered under the weight of dozens of unpaid parking tickets—I thought, *Fuck it*, and never saw it again. Later, during my first real job, at Morgan Stanley, I was given the profoundly complex task of hand-delivering a proposal to a client. All I had to do was board an a.m. flight to San Francisco. I missed the flight.

Among other things, the brain's prefrontal cortex helps us get the easy stuff right. Until twenty-five, I got more than my fair share of easy stuff wrong, didn't take responsibility, most of the time had no ability to plan, and continually messed up.

A tendency for risk-taking, mixed with poor impulse control, renders many young men helpless against a torrent of on-demand dopamine provided by the world's richest tech companies and makes maturity a hard sell for teen- and college-age boys—at least, relative to girls and young women. You almost never hear about people named Laura and Elena eating Tide Pods or blowing off their final exams. Why?

Male and female brains are more than 99 percent identical. There are variations, though. Men have more than double the brain space and processing power devoted to sexual drive. The male amygdala, home to fear, anger, and aggression, contains testosterone receptors that make males lose their cool faster and more easily. But where the male and female brains diverge most sharply is in their development, especially during adolescence. By age fourteen to sixteen, male and female brains have stopped growing, with the exception of the prefrontal cortex, or PFC. Girls attain "peak values of brain volumes" earlier than boys do—Latin for "girls get their shit together way sooner." Basically, the female PFC matures up to two years before the male PFC does.

The PFC is the grown-up in the room, the CEO. The brain is a network; e.g., overlap is a feature, not a bug. No single brain region governs one instinct. But science agrees that a healthy PFC regulates impulse control, decision-making, good judgment, reasonableness, emotional regulation, and planning/prioritizing between the stuff you have to do versus the stuff you'd rather be doing (getting drunk or high, rewatching *Family Guy*).

At the start of puberty, boys are basically marinated in testosterone. T makes them more monosyllabic than usual. Their socializing, never strong to begin with, narrows to sports/physical activity, depending on the kid, and thinking about sex. With their thicker, denser muscles and deeper voices, boys may look impressive and imposing, but behind the forehead, girls have lapped them. By fourteen to fifteen, girls have greater volume and complexity in their PFCs and thus, theoretically, more maturity than boys. They're better decision-makers and problem-solvers. They can overcome their brains' reward circuits with a good counterargument or simply by deploying common sense.

The male PFC catches up around age twenty-five, when many young men get their act together. Until then, they're at a huge maturity disadvantage.

The schism between male chronological age and brain age is one reason why, along with their higher likelihood to be diagnosed with ADHD and autism, and with the dearth of male teachers in all phases of their education, boys fall behind academically early on and often never catch up. Note: diagnostic bias also plays a part, with studies showing that ADHD in girls is more likely to be overlooked than in boys, and that white kids from higher socioeconomic backgrounds

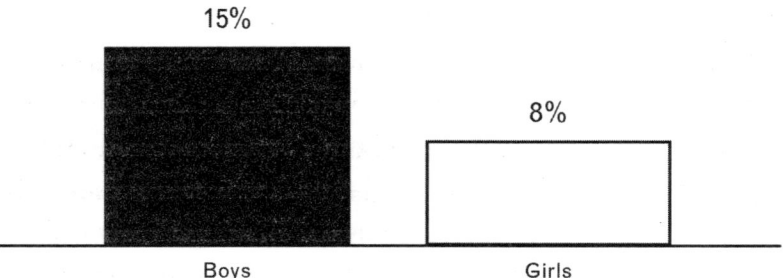

Share of Children Ever Diagnosed with ADHD
U.S., 2022, Children Aged 3–17

Boys: 15%
Girls: 8%

Source: U.S. Centers for Disease Control.

are in general identified with ASD (autism spectrum disorder) earlier than Black, Latino, and Asian children, along with kids from underprivileged families. As to whether the absence of male educators affects academic outcomes, the evidence is inconclusive, according to Richard Reeves. It's why he has proposed redshirting boys in high school, to delay their enrollment in college for a year.

Waging war against a young man's unformed PFC is like trying to wean a kid off salty snacks in favor of carrots and radishes. With my two boys, I do my best to illustrate the differences between the feverish, relentless dopa hits they get from TikTok and Instagram versus the slower, incremental results that are more valuable and satisfying from reading, working out, or spending time outside—slow dopa, or "Slowpa," as I call it. If tech dopa hits are like shoving endless handfuls of Cheetos or Snickers into your mouth—i.e., they don't fill you up, you hate yourself, and you want more—Slowpa more closely resembles the salad you order that makes you feel healthier for a week.

When my boys were little, we spent a fortune on LEGOs. If Slowpa ever hires a celebrity spokesperson, it should be LEGO. Building a model out of thirteen hundred pieces of lightly hued plastic requires one to two hours daily, plus focus, but then two weeks later you have a really cool Millennium Falcon or Blacktron Renegade to hang in your bedroom.

Sometimes Slowpa happens organically. On weekends, my oldest son, Alec, likes to cook with his mom. They spend two hours chopping and prepping, the dish goes into the oven for an hour and/or sits out overnight until it's ready to eat—delayed gratification; i.e., Slowpa.

Children today are overprotected in the real world and underprotected online—an observation made by my NYU colleague Jonathan Haidt. At age thirteen, I flew from LAX alone to visit my dad and stepmom in Ohio. Looking back, the 1970s may seem lax, negligent, and flaky, but parents were onto something. Nowadays, if, say, my fourteen-year-old son wants to have a party, no, I won't go out and score a case of tequila for him, but I won't hover, snoop, or get in the way of his plans, either.

Last year, Nolan, my youngest, was having trouble waking up and getting out of bed in the morning. My wife and I decided to butt out—it was his problem, not ours, and he was too old for his mom to tiptoe in at six thirty a.m. to rouse him. For two weeks, Nolan slept in, showed up late to school, and was marked tardy. It happened so many times the school told him he couldn't accompany his classmates on a big field trip to Ireland. He'd really been looking forward to it. "You blew it," I said. These days, he sets his phone alarm the night before.

Recently, he made a plan to meet some school friends at a mall. I arranged an Uber, but the Uber dropped him off at the wrong mall. Panicked, Nolan texted us. To be clear, it was my fault, and my wife was minorly pissed. But if I'd responded to my son's texts by freaking out, it would have taught him to panic in any situation that isn't scripted, lubricated, or minutely staged and choreographed by his parents. He had a smartphone and an Uber account, so I texted him: *You've got this, figure it out.* He did. It made him feel good, too.

In sum, my wife and I do our best not to track our boys. It's healthier for them, and for us, not knowing where they are all the time.

I recently showed both boys a TikTok by some ex–finance guy. What he said was basic, obvious, and great: success comes when you put in small, consistent amounts of effort, every day and every week; it doesn't matter whether you're investing, filming two minutes of video content, or lifting dumbbells. Small, deliberate, regular efforts accumulate and in time pay off. In other words, the most powerful force in the universe—Einstein knew this but kept his mouth shut—is compound interest. Slowpa.

Note: *Success comes when you put in small, consistent amounts of effort, every day and every week.*

chapter 2

THINGS GET HAIRY: ADOLESCENCE

THE WEATHER UP THERE

When I say I peaked at age eight or nine, I'm not exaggerating. I had a few flashes of potential greatness, but so do most kids. I never stood out. If you're still unconvinced, the state school in my neighborhood, twelve blocks from our apartment, had a 76 percent admissions rate. They rejected me.

Puberty, and a growth spurt unaccompanied by weight gain, blessed me seemingly overnight with the height of a thirteen-year-old and the strength and coordination of a nine-year-old. I went from being a robust, strong kid to a tall, skinny, underpowered kid. Other boys, better favored by testosterone, were morphing into amazing physical specimens, whereas my own gross motor skills couldn't keep up with my suddenly dangling arms and stilt-like legs. I'd developed acne, too, not terrible but bad enough. I could no longer compete athletically with my peers. I was also now attending a bigger, integrated school, Emerson. I had a classmate who, in eighth grade, could dunk a basketball. My two best friends' parents pulled them from Emerson to send them to a nearby private school instead. I stayed put.

My drift into unremarkableness continued. Not excelling at anything, few friends, no real sense of self. Invisible. Scott the Friendly Ghost. My grades were all B's and C's, and I didn't test well, either. No teachers, skilled at pattern recognition and sensing my infinite potential, took me under their wing. In eighth grade, I was downgraded from Calculus to Algebra 2, then Algebra 1. I just couldn't figure it out. I ran for junior, sophomore, and senior class student body president and lost all three times. I was also cut from JV baseball. Basically, I was a mediocre kid (being generous) at a mediocre high school (again, generous) in Santa Monica, surrounded by kids who used to steal cocaine from their parents and race their parents' cars on Sunset Boulevard. Not so much *Fast & Furious* as Lame & Entitled. The only remarkable thing about me was my willingness to endure repeated failure.

Body image issues aren't just for women. Boys have them, too. Body dysmorphia, as it's called, is a serious psychiatric condition. Male sufferers are preoccupied with an imagined and offending body part: their ears, their noses, their butts, their dicks. They can spend hours every day grooming, checking their reflection repeatedly in the mirror, and camouflaging the body parts they hate the most. One study reported that 10 to 30 percent of American men are dissatisfied with their bodies, with nearly 70 percent of all adolescent males unhappy with their weight, and nearly 90 percent with their musculature.

More than body dysmorphia, I probably had one of its subsets—muscle dysmorphia. I was insecure about my body and my build. I disliked my body and what it couldn't do. I felt too weak, too skinny, too un-virile.

Genetics influenced my build, but environment played a part, too. In my household, food wasn't nutrition; it was punishment. At home, it was just the two of us, my mom was stretched thin, and we didn't have a lot of money. So every Sunday afternoon she would prepare a huge vat of shepherd's pie. Potatoes, corn, and beef, under an overcast lid of more mashed potatoes. We had it for dinner, and that first night it tasted fine, even good.

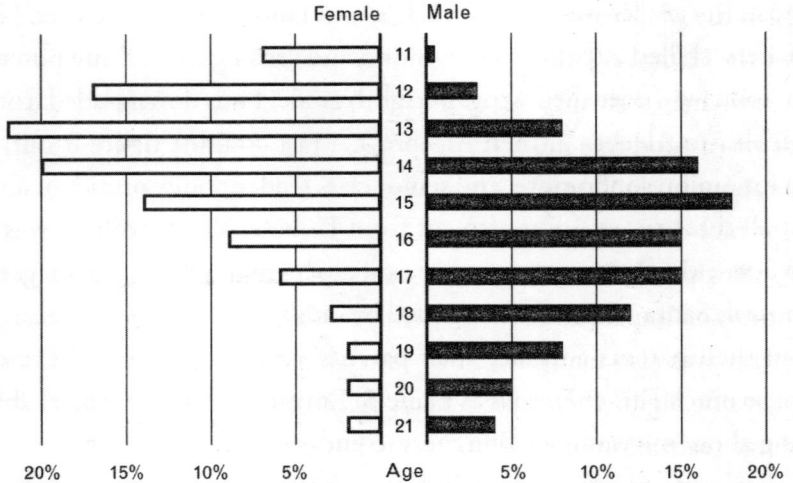

Age of Onset of Body Dysmorphia
U.S., by Gender, 2022

Source: Suzanna Diaz and J. Michael Bailey, "Rapid Onset Gender Dysphoria: Parent Reports on 1,655 Possible Cases," *Archives of Sexual Behavior* 52, no. 3 (April 2023): 1031–43.

My mom would then cut the shepherd's pie into eight individual slabs and freeze them. That was my menu for the week. I would come home, forage for a slab, and stick it in the microwave. Microwaving back then was a primitive technology. During the countdown, it sounded like a boardwalk reunion of the Hells Angels, or Chernobyl about to blow. When the bell sounded, I would remove this wet, gross chunk of shepherd's pie and force it down my throat. It was like shoveling dirt into a burial plot, a labor, completely non-sensory.

A SAVING GRACE

Downgraded to Algebra 1 in eighth grade, only later did I do the emotional math. When my dad left, so did a male role model. Coincidence or not, my life started going downhill for me when my dad left.

Terry helped.

My mom now had a boyfriend. Terry was a nice man and always generous to us. He and my mom were together for ten years. He gave her the money to buy a condo in Westwood, a much nicer neighborhood, and a big upgrade from Tarzana. More than that, he was fully engaged in the well-being of his girlfriend's son (me). This was in the days before the Catholic Church and Michael Jackson fucked up the concept of a grown man showing interest in a boy's development and well-being. Terry was a good role model for me—an entrepreneur who would talk to me about business, a handsome, well-dressed guy who would take us out for nice dinners and tip the staff generously. He spent every other weekend with us. He made our lives tangibly better. I learned, firsthand, the profound impact an older man can have on a younger man's life.

Terry was also married, with a school-age son. My mom blurted this out one night when she and Terry were briefly on the outs. It was a strange realization to have in my forties that when I was a kid, I was in some man's "other" family. Movies and TV shows are never about the second family and focus instead on the wreckage visited on the first. The knee-jerk response: This is a bad dude. Terry wasn't. When I heard about his other family, I remember thinking, *Life is complicated.*

I WAS ALSO PREPARED . . .

The Boy Scouts also saved me from utter obscurity. The Scouts was a safe place for me and other kids "in the middle." We were (mostly) not the high achievers academically or (definitely not) the cool kids. Just . . . well . . . boys in the middle. We were exposed to the outdoors and gained confidence there, hiking with a heavy pack, taking some of the load off other patrol members. We learned to respect nature, scouring the campground before we left to cleanse it of any litter or evidence we had been there. Mostly, though, the Scouts were about camaraderie and community. While not an Eagle, I earned several merit badges, including the Fire Safety badge. To this day, every hotel I check into I register a mental map of the hallway and exits, and plan my escape on my hands and knees with a dampened towel over my mouth. I wore my uniform to school every Wednesday—something my best friend from home announces whenever we're in a group setting.

Robert Baden-Powell, the former British army officer and rumored spy who founded the Boy Scouts in the early twentieth century, was raised, as I was, by a strong mother. His own dad died when he was three. He gave his mom credit for everything. *Be Prepared* doubles as his initials. It also meant he expected boys to be in a constant state of readiness, in mind and body, to do their duty, whatever it might be. Great advice for men of any age.

BENJAMINS

Starting when I was young, money was a constant theme. My high school was racially and economically diverse—a third Black kids, 20 percent Latino, and the rest of the student body white. These days, every wealthy kid in L.A. attends a private school, but back then, some rich kids still went the public route. I was never self-conscious about not having money, but at some point it became clear that my mom and I were different because we didn't have any. Basically, if you were white, and living in Westwood, as we were, you were supposed to have money. If you didn't, something was wrong—probably you.

People who don't grow up with economic constraints have no idea what it's like. Not having money is like being followed around all day by a wispy capitalist ghost. I felt this ghost follow me to school every day, and tuck in beside me at night. The ghost wouldn't shut up. It whispered in my ear that my mom and I had fucked up, we were failures. That I shouldn't reach for much educationally, professionally, romantically. That I couldn't even attend the 7:10 movie showing, because the nighttime ticket cost three bucks more than the matinee. In America, how much money you have or don't have seems like the only benchmark that matters. In time, worn down, I began trusting the ghost and believing it was a spokesperson for the whole country. Eventually, the ghost started to piss me off. *Okay,* I told myself, *if*

America is all about money, I want some. The modern analogy is social media that reminds young people they're falling behind some impossible standard. *You don't have a six-pack? You didn't make three million dollars trading dojo coin? You're not staying at the Aman Resort in Utah or the Yellowstone Club in Montana?* America is world class as a shamemaker. It provoked something deep and relentless in me.

I used to visit my two best friends, Adam and David, at their tony nearby private school, Windward. The campus was a snow globe, cozy and insular. In biology class, Adam and David went on a field trip scuba diving off Catalina Island. Needless to say, scuba diving wasn't a thing at Emerson. That night, I told my mom I needed to go to Windward, too. It was a "moment," and there were a few, when my mom sat me down and told me that we—I—couldn't do X and Y because we just didn't have the money.

The same thing happened at Hebrew school. The first two classes—no problem. The people there were kind and welcoming. This evolved into *We need to speak to your mom.* I remember that phone conversation, as it was clearly a money call. *Why do you want to go to Hebrew school?* my mom asked after she hung up. *Why do you need to be Bar Mitzvahed?* I couldn't come up with an answer aside from the fact my friends were doing it. Again, she told me we were—I was—different. We—I—couldn't afford Hebrew school. She could have told the school that, and they would have probably figured something out. But when you grow up without money, you lack even the confidence to consider making that call.

At the time, I wanted money for a more pedestrian purpose: to buy a car. It was my primary focus from the ages of eleven to sixteen. By sixteen, I'd saved $2,000. By freshman year in college, it was up to $3,000. My mom never once asked me to reallocate that money toward household expenses. She knew that a disproportionate amount of a boy's manhood in Los Angeles is connected to his wheels.

A current trend among Gen Z is scrapping this rite of passage by delaying getting a driver's license. Ride-sharing is a big factor behind this, as are the costs of owning, maintaining, and insuring a car. In 1997, approximately 90 percent of twenty- to twenty-five-year-olds had licenses. By 2020, this had fallen 10 percentage points. For young people, getting a driver's license has developmental ramifications: they're free, behind the wheel, literally and metaphorically; they're accountable; and they're tasked with navigating potential life-or-death scenarios (crowded highways, drunk drivers). My oldest son, Alec, was fifteen when he took a test online, did a few hours of driving school, and was given his Florida learner's permit. He drove us home, at one point stopping at a red light. When, a few seconds later, he pulled into the intersection to make a left turn, I began screaming. With eerie professional calm, my son said, "Dad, I'm allowed to make a left on a red light as long as I come to a stop first." I screamed louder.

I believe parents should encourage kids to take risks, learn, fuck up, scrape the garage door, drive into a trellis, get a flat tire, develop accountability, and manage the costs of driving. Driving helps young people calibrate; e.g., *I've had two beers so I shouldn't drive; I'll leave the car at my friend's and take an Uber; The insurance payment is due.* The ability to handle a car, parallel park, and vary your speed is a dumb but easy way to demonstrate male excellence and the ability to protect

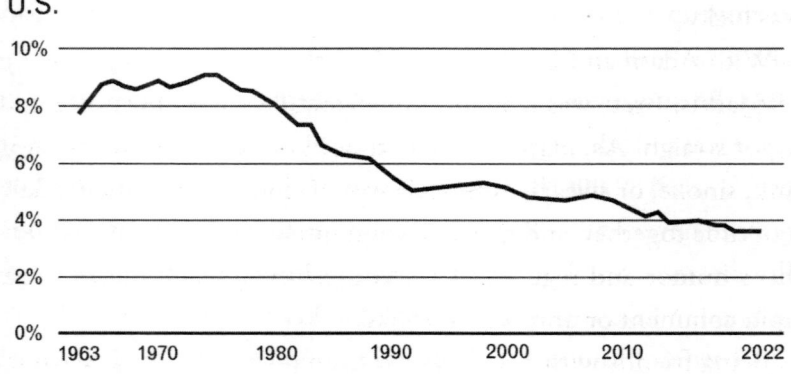

Drivers Age 19 and Under as a Share of Total Drivers
U.S.

Source: U.S. Dept. of Transportation.

others. I'm trying to convince my son to drive cross-country with his best friend before college. There'll be some weird spots, possibly a horrific learning experience or two, but it's good preparation for life. Knowing she'll freak out, I haven't mentioned this idea yet to his mom.

At fifteen, I got my learner's permit. My mom and I would practice driving in the garage. Home from work, she would honk her horn as she entered the garage below our apartment complex, signaling for me to come down and practice, on inclines in the massive garage, how to drive a stick shift.

When I turned sixteen, she drove up in a four-year-old BMW 320i and gave me the keys to her eight-year-old Opel Manta. She put the keys in my hands, rested her hands (up) on my shoulders, and said, "You're a handsome young man [I wasn't] who owns his own car." I've bought, and been given, a lot of nice things. This stands alone as the most joyous moment I've registered from an inanimate object.

PEER REVIEW

We parents believe we can engineer our kids, but we're more like shepherds. We choose where our children graze, what foods they eat, and where they sleep. We can angle them in the right direction. Our godlike power and impact end there. In terms of influence, dwarfing parents are the peers a high school kid hangs out with. In that sense, I was lucky.

With Adam and David gone, my best friend in high school was Brett Jarvis. Brett was from an upper-middle-class Mormon family. He got straight A's, played on the school basketball team, and didn't drink, smoke, or swear—even soda was off-limits. Brett and I spent a lot of time together, and he was a good influence on me. We got each other's humor and regularly found ourselves in hysterics over some stupid comment or unrepeatable joke.

Being friends with Brett was protective—best friend as talisman. At home I had almost no parental supervision and, apart from Terry, no male role models. Yet as a sixteen-year-old, I was impressionable. If I'd hung out with boys who jacked cars or were permanently wasted, I would have likely gone down some dusky, belligerent path. Instead, every Monday night I went over to the Jarvis house for a convivial sit-down dinner. Nothing mattered more to Brett's parents than family. His mom and dad were basically unpaid Uber drivers, shepherding their sons to various lessons, practices, events, and games. Since Brett didn't drink or smoke weed, I didn't, either. Being as I was a somewhat lazy, underachieving kid, my friendship with Brett pushed me to focus on classes and sports more than was probably my natural inclination. Brett was on his way to Stanford. He had a clear plan—and so college was folded into mine.

Another good friend was Drew Sheldon, who was smart, confident, and funny. Drew was a Black boy from downtown L.A. who got bused into Emerson post-integration. At six-foot-two, 195 pounds, and all muscle, he played middle linebacker on the varsity football team. Though not a great student, he was blessed with social skills and charm. The most impressive thing about Drew, in my eyes, was that he was having more sex with more girls than anyone I'd ever met. As I was still a virgin, I found this hard to relate to, but that didn't mean I didn't salivate hearing his stories about late nights and cheerleaders.

The Emerson football team played games on Friday nights. On the second play of one game, Drew pinched a nerve in his neck and had to leave the field. I found him on the sidelines, where an ambulance always hovered, as high school football players are at high risk of getting injured. "Is Drew going to be okay?" I asked one of the EMTs. "He'll be fine," one said.

It didn't explain why Drew was sitting there, his chest heaving, sobbing. I'd never seen a boy my age crying like that. That Friday night, it turned out, was the one time a year football scouts showed up at our school on the lookout for promising recruits. "I'm not going to college," Drew sobbed.

It was the first time I was aware that a person's good fortune and position in life is relative. I'd always been insecure about my family's economic situation. Always cognizant my dad was gone and my mom worked as a secretary. I was never self-pitying, but felt I could have been dealt a better hand. Still, the landing lights were always on for me to go to college. For Drew, the math was different. He was an okay student; that's all. His family—they lived in Hancock Park, his larger-than-life dad a minister with a booming voice—didn't have much money. Without a sports scholarship, Drew's future was in play. A football snap and a compressed nerve root was all it took.

Whenever I talk about young men online, many readers leave comments along the lines of "Oh, poor white men." This is a mischaracterization—the issues and challenges young men are facing are especially acute among young men of color. A boy or young man in general of any race is twice as likely to get suspended from school than his female equivalent, whereas a Black boy is five times as likely. In 2019, 28 percent of Black men ages twenty-five to twenty-nine had a BA or higher, versus 30 percent of Black women and more than 40 percent of white men. Black workers of both genders earn less than white workers, including white women, and labor force participation for Black men aged twenty and over is nearly 6 percent lower than it is for white men. As of 2021, Black youth were 4.7 times more likely to be placed in juvenile facilities than their white peers, and as of 2010, Black men were over six times as likely as white men to be incarcerated in prison or jail, and Hispanic men were three times as likely. On average, Black men also die four years earlier than white men.

Drew may have been funny, charming, and jacked, but his opportunity set was already narrowing. *Everyone has problems*, I remember thinking, *and some people have it worse than me*. It didn't matter how big, strong, and seemingly invincible Drew was. His physical prowess and track record with women had nothing to do with his ability to handle problems or navigate his own future. That night, Drew was vulnerable and scared. His popularity, coolness, and athleticism couldn't fix the rest of his life.

I may have been unrelentingly unremarkable in high school, and I can't say I retained much of what I was taught, but I did absorb a few lessons. From hanging out with Brett's family, I had learned to appreciate the presence of a strong, loving, dependable support system. Unbeknownst to him, and along with his cheerleader stories, Drew now left me with something else. As cool and good with girls as he was, college was now off the table for him because the one night a year when football scouts showed up at Emerson, he had the bad luck to pinch a nerve in his neck. Seeing him there on the sidelines, I was overcome with empathy. Compared with that of some kids, no, my situation wasn't great, but compared with others it was good enough. Some incidents, like that one, usher in a wave of growing up, though mostly I felt for Drew, my friend.

High school ended, and Drew and I lost touch—I wish we hadn't. After graduating Stanford, Brett went to the Kellogg School of Management and worked a series of tech jobs. Today he lives in Utah, has three kids, has been happily married for thirty years, still goes to church every Sunday, is a wonderful husband and father, and lives an incredibly rewarding life. Nothing surprises me less.

THE SORTING HAT

Put a bunch of humans in a room or school and it's scary how fast groups and hierarchies form. School is the first time kids are ranked, sidelined, and/or sanctified. Adolescence is a caste system based not on who your family is, as in Europe, but on good looks, great bodies, and money. The hierarchies vary based on when and where you grow up, but they're also disconcertingly fixed.

At the bottom of the ladder at Emerson were boys who were awkward and struggling. Today, we would diagnose them and get them help, but back then they were just weird and dorky. A rung or two up were the artsy, alternative kids. From a popularity standpoint, they functioned at the same angle indie bands did to classic rock. Rejecting the era's coolness standards, they sought shelter in their own cultish unconformity. I was good friends with two kids from the drama club, David Bowe and Andy Lauer, both edgy, popular, funny, and rambunctious. They both ended up going into show business and had some early success on TV and in movies, but unless you're Clint Eastwood, that industry sucks.

At the pinnacle of high school capital were the boys—now young men—who'd matured before the rest of us. The same third shot of testosterone that stretched my body out to gumlike proportions had ushered them into confident future versions of themselves. Exit cuteness, enter handsomeness. Facial and body hair aside, testosterone worked for them as it hadn't for me, granting them bigger muscles, deeper voices, confident coordination, and more aggression. They weren't unkind, just mildly combative. Other boys wanted to be friends with them, and girls wanted to flirt with and sleep with them. They had evolved into procreators, at the mercy and pleasure of their own undeveloped prefrontal cortices (impulse largely unbothered by forethought).

In high school, the chances of me procreating were the same as me becoming fourth in line to the British throne. No girl expressed any desire to have sex with me, and if she had, (a) I would have been too dumb and immature to realize it, and (b) it would have freaked me out.

Harder to identify in this taxonomy were boys like Brett and me. We were cool-adjacent—never allowed membership in the actual cool crowd but granted an occasional visitor's pass. I would hear about weekend parties I wasn't invited to and crash them. The other kids were fine with me being there, hospitable even—no one ever beat me up or hog-tied me with rope or threw me into a pool and watched me sink. Sometimes I would even hang out with an actual cool kid. It's probably confirmation bias, but being cool-adjacent is not a bad goal for teenagers. It's incredibly motivating. A lot of kids who were cool in high school crash and flame out by the age of thirty. When life gets hard, or they're faced with their first disappointment, many don't know what to do and flounder. Whereas if you're near-cool, like Brett and me, and punching above your weight class, there's always something to shoot for.

Studies show that women are generally attracted to men for three reasons. Number three is kindness, number two is intellect, and number one is resources (not just money per se but also ambition, social status, and the potential for career success: Can you take care of potential offspring?). I had no resources to speak of. My parents didn't own a house in Aspen or Palm Springs, my dad wasn't an agent or the head of a movie studio, and I didn't drive a BMW convertible. Kindness didn't register on my radar back then—that would take me a while. Early on I figured out that whatever social capital I possessed would be based on humor; i.e., telling clever, goofy stories. Wit may be a Freudian defense mechanism, but it works and also signals intellect. Make a girl laugh, and she might hang out with me. Keep the jokes coming, and she might let me kiss her or even sleep with her. That was the Dadaist fantasy at least.

In ninth grade, I was voted "most comical." And "Steve Martin." Not "Most Like Steve Martin," just "Steve Martin." This wasn't random. Steve Martin was America's first arena-rock comedian, and everyone at school had one or both of his albums. In contrast to my lesser role models—John Travolta, who danced and fought in *Saturday Night Fever*; Harrison Ford playing Han Solo; and various musicians in vogue, like Billy Joel, Elton John, and Ric Ocasek of the Cars—what reputation I had in high school bore, in spirit, Steve Martin's chalky complexion and ghost hair.

Wit is different from charm. In fact, being offensive—the opposite of charm—is something I later developed a knack for. Saying things at the worst possible time. Even in my thirties, I used to regularly say things and write emails that made good people feel bad, and I knew it. Whether it was a defense mechanism or me just being a dick, well, trust your instincts. But a sense of humor planted the seeds in me of being a decent storyteller, which was in my DNA anyway, thanks to my sometimes incorrigible dad.

WHY DON'T YOU DO RIGHT?

Beer, weed, tobacco—most substances held no appeal for me in high school. Again, being friends with Brett, a Mormon, and Drew, an athlete, saved me from any worst-case scenarios.

My parents were lifelong heavy smokers—my dad, Marlboros; my mom, Salems. I have an old photo of my mom with a drink in one hand and a cigarette in the other when she was eight months pregnant with me. Once, before the divorce, I had such a vicious cough, I had to go to the doctor. This was so alien and cinematic an excursion that both my mom and dad came along. I was diagnosed with a serious lung infection, and the doctor forbade my parents to smoke around me during my recovery. Yeah, sure. My dad drove home with all the car windows cranked open to let the smoke flutter out. At home, he wet a towel and half-rolled, half-jammed it under my bedroom door so he and my mom could puff away unbothered.

These days, I'm almost never sick. I've missed work maybe two or three days in the past four decades. I credit this to never seeing a doctor or getting antibiotics when I was a kid. Harvard should study me.

Another drug popular in the 1970s was cocaine. Many of my classmates' parents were in the entertainment industry. On the weekends, they would disappear to their second homes, leaving behind their kids, mini-Gatsbys who threw riotous parties. Everyone would show up and snort Mom and Dad's blow. As a kid, I was once kicked in the face during youth soccer, the result being that once or twice a week, usually in the middle of the night, my nose would begin spraying blood. My mom would come in, sit patiently by my side, and level my head. To calm me, she and I would do math problems together, since I always liked math. The bleeding would stop, and I'd fall asleep. I knew enough to realize it probably wasn't smart to develop a cocaine habit, given my habit of spewing blood out of my nose.

But the biggest factor behind my not getting regularly drunk or high was my family situation. It wasn't like I was a great son who devoted his days to helping out his single mom. Like most teens, I went through a period when I wasn't very nice to her—rolling my eyes, dissing her. Kids need to do this—deciding your parents are lame is preparation for leaving—but it makes me sad to remember.

If the three tenets of being a man are to protect, provide, and procreate, the last two were beyond my reach. This left protection. I did this the only way I could—by recognizing that my mom couldn't have handled having a son who got into trouble. During my friends' shoplifting excursions, I would wait outside while they busily stuffed T-shirts, posters, and record albums into their shirts and pants. Not because I was more ethical than them, but because I knew if my mom got a call from the West L.A. police department asking her to pick up her son, she couldn't have handled it. My mom was fragile after the divorce, often on the verge of tears if not hysteria about money and other concerns. *I am not going to bring this shit into our house*, I thought, this shit being my misbehavior. Maybe I wasn't a kid a parent could boast about, who threw touchdowns or brought home character awards, but I wasn't about to wreak more havoc in her life.

BOY PLANET

A lot has changed since I was in high school, but American boy culture, though kinder and more demonstrative today—boys and men hug more these days—is mostly fixed. Lots of unspoken mandates: Play sports. Make fun of your friends. Possibly get into a scrap or two. When I was in high school, karate was popular, and many of my friends went to dojos. Better to be a boy who broke boards with his hands than an academic grinder. The most admired boy in my class was Luke

Guilfoyle. He would fight anyone and win. He was also irrepressible and obnoxious. One day during lunch he came over to a table where I was sitting with three other guys. He unzipped his jeans and pulled out his hard-on. *Watch it move*, Luke commanded, and we looked on as it flexed and bobbed. It was both horrifying and impressive.

Our favorite activity was breaking into the school building after dark. We did this roughly once a week. We weren't being criminal, just sneaky. Once we were inside, what did we do? Not much. We roamed around like crap ninjas. Entered and exited classrooms. Someone might leave the premises with a few rolls of toilet paper under his shirt. My friends and I hated school during the day when we had to be there. When we didn't, there was literally no place on earth more magical.

As for being a good student—there was some prestige to that among boys. Every year, there seemed to be two boys and two girls who were unusually smart. The girls were always well rounded and impressive. You got the sense with the boys that they would remain virgins for a long time. (Intelligence may be a desirable trait in men, but it likely depends on what kind.) But intelligence wasn't grounds for exclusion, given the Space Race, after all. Smarts could take you to Houston, and NASA, where you could build rockets, possibly end up on the moon.

Walking from Westwood Village back home, I crossed Hilgard Avenue, where UCLA sororities lined the street. It was homecoming week, and there were thousands of young women standing in front of their houses, singing songs and generally looking like a cross between a Norman Rockwell painting and a late-night Cinemax movie. Then and there, I decided I would attend UCLA.

SHELVED, BRIEFLY

My dad had other plans for me. He always hoped I would do better than him, though he was never willing to sacrifice to make that happen.

In my senior year of high school, he took me on a tour of the Naval Academy in Annapolis. Because he had served in the Royal

Navy, it made complete sense to him that I should attend Annapolis. If I got in, he told me, he'd even buy me a Trans Am. This was another touching snapshot of parental naivete. I was an okay student, if that. The kids who get into Annapolis are strong academically as well as incredibly impressive and disciplined. A personal nomination from either a senator, member of the House, or military serviceperson is also mandatory. I had access to none of those. It was like taking Spicoli, the Sean Penn character from *Fast Times at Ridgemont High*, to the doors of MIT and demanding a sit-down with the provost. Not going to happen. I didn't apply. I set my sights instead on UCLA.

UCLA rejected me, which didn't seem like a big deal—my father assured me that "someone with your street smarts doesn't need college." Uh, I had no street smarts, just a father with a new family who didn't want to pay for college. My dad did, however, find me a job installing shelving. I'd get into my car and drive an hour and go into a closet for eighteen bucks an hour. At the time, it felt like a lot of money, though in its disfavor was working inside a closet. The only thing I looked forward to was getting ridiculously high with my coworkers and driving the Southern California freeways.

I had no other options for college, and getting into UCLA would mean I could continue to live at home with my mom. One day, I broke down in front of her. *Everyone has always said I'm smart and funny*, I said. *Now I'm going to be working inside a closet for the rest of my life*. No, there was and is nothing wrong with trade work—it just didn't match the expectations I'd built up and others had given me.

Is there anything we can do? My mom, the problem solver. Yes. There was an appeal process. It involved writing a one-page letter. I sent it in, and nine days before classes started in September, the phone rang. UCLA had reviewed my transcript, and despite my mediocre grades and SAT scores, they were letting me in, as I was "a son of a single mother and the great state of California" (no joke, those were the exact words). *We're going to give you a shot.*

I remember my mom and me going to Junior's Deli to celebrate. She told me that, as the first person to attend college on either side of the family, I could now "do anything." As my options were now limitless, I committed to spending the next five years smoking a shit-ton of pot (pretty much everyone in my fraternity smoked; it was contagious), playing sports, and watching the *Planet of the Apes* trilogy several dozen times, taking breaks from this routine only for random sexual encounters. Except for the last part, I was hugely successful.

Still, it was the start of an upward spiral. Today, we hold on to the notion that inner-city neighborhoods are quietly teeming with undiscovered, remarkable, unburnished jewels. The Ivy League says it wants to go into these communities and pull those people out. It's not that easy.

When you're poor and born to unsophisticated parents, and you get the message early on that having no money means you and your family are unworthy to the point that you start believing it, how do you even take the first step? When UCLA turned me down the first time, I remember someone said, *Well then, why don't you go to UMich or someplace like that?* The University of Michigan might as well have been the University of Mars. We just didn't have the money. I didn't have a credit card. I didn't know how to buy a plane ticket or reserve a hotel room or arrange an interview or even what to wear. People born and raised in middle- or upper-income homes take so much for granted in terms of their inborn skills, cultural knowledge, connections, and confidence. It's not just a lack of economic wherewithal; it's a lack of worldliness, self-worth, and deservingness. Growing up without money shrinks your sense of what's within reach. I could have applied to CalState Northridge, but I assumed getting rejected by UCLA meant the entire university ecosystem had foreclosed on my future; i.e., smart people believed I wasn't college material. (I'd also missed the CalState application deadline.) Eighteen bucks an hour to work in a closet was, for me, a pretty decent deal. In my head, I was either going to UCLA or I would spend the rest of my life putting up shelves.

Once, not terribly long ago, America loved the unremarkable. *Do you want to take some chances?* it asked. *A risk or two? Do you have talent? Skills? Drive?* We would then give the people who said yes the opportunity to blossom maybe later in life instead of identifying who is already remarkable at sixteen or seventeen and putting even more pressure on them to shock and awe us. Again, no organization or person or university can or should be the arbiter of any young person's projected success. You never know when someone will decode the puzzle of himself and bloom. The goal, it seems to me, is to plant as much soil and as many nutrients around as many seeds as possible, as opposed to force-watering a few already half-ripened super-seeds and tending them in a hydroponic bubble, and good luck to all the others who are left untended to dry, wilt, turn to powder, and blow away. Today, the American koan goes something like this: Let's identify a super class of freakishly remarkable, prematurely accomplished young people and see if we can't sculpt them into billionaires. Versus giving as many young people as possible a decent shot at becoming millionaires or finding various versions of success.

THE POWER OF KINDNESS

Looking back, the only reason I got into UCLA was because of one teacher. Ms. Kelson was her name. She taught high school biology. Around school she was known as a hard-ass who took unseemly pride in doling out only a handful of A's every year. She was a good teacher, though neither popular nor likable. Older, heavyset, scowling, with a thick accent and an office desk adorned with photos of her many cats. But I liked her, and I liked biology, too.

In my senior year of high school, when Valentine's Day came, I bought Ms. Kelson a giant chocolate bar. Probably a 100 Grand bar, which Nestlé no longer makes, which I probably bought for 79 cents at the bargain bin at our local Gemco. The chocolate bar was ridiculously large, the size of a human head. I left it on Ms. Kelson's desk, anonymously, tied with a ribbon. I don't know how she found out it was from me, but she did.

I worked my ass off in biology, and Ms. Kelson gave me an A. Why? Because I was kind to her. I didn't expect the gift of a giant chocolate bar to influence my final grade; no one, except for whoever told her I'd left it there, saw me enter her office. When UCLA reconsidered my admission, the admission person who let me in brought up my A in biology. Ms. Kelson's reputation was sterling. Getting an A from her had meaning.

Did I deserve it? I'll never know. But at that moment I realized that kindness pays off, especially when it's directed at a person who probably wasn't used to getting much.

Kindness would save me a second time at UCLA. In my senior year in college, I was on the verge of not graduating, having failed calculus twice. If I retook and failed calculus a third time, UCLA wouldn't allow me to take it again. Lights out for me. I would have to change my major from economics to psychology, which meant spending two more years in college, or six in all, and I didn't have the money to do that.

I went to the professor's office. I can't remember his name, but what I do remember is how overworked he was—there must have been four hundred kids in the class. Taking a seat, I pleaded my case. I told him I was in trouble, that I'd gotten a job offer from Morgan Stanley that was conditional on my graduating from college. By then I was back living at home with my mom, and I had to get out of there.

The professor could have said *Tough* or some variation of *Shit happens*. He didn't. Instead, he took the time to sit down beside me and go over a bunch of concepts. He made sure I was at least conversant with the material. He told me to come back the following day with some problem sets. I did, and we worked through those, too. He did this for two, three days straight. I wasn't sure where this was going, but when it was over, he told me it was obvious to him I had a fundamental understanding of calculus. He gave me a B, which, however undeserved, was more than enough for me to pass.

It's probably one reason why I entered academia—a lot of decent people work there. Deep down, most people (including, believe it or not, me) are good. They're looking for opportunities to help others out.

Kindness and asking for help are two unheralded weapons for men. They're big components of being male, and both go a long way. Unfortunately, many boys and men never figure this out.

Note: *Be kind. Ask for help. Model yourself on— learn from—the people who've helped you.*

WHAT A DIFFERENCE A GENERATION MAKES

A few years ago, my family and I were at the tail end of a two-week ski trip that had gone on a week too long. We were in Courchevel, France, which is a bad Aspen, and, along with golf, I hate skiing. (There, I said it. I'm pretty sure—and hoping—that both won't exist in fifty years.) However, each year we would put our boys on skis so they could become competent skiers and so, when they were teenagers, we could entrap them for several hours on a mountain and force them to spend time with us.

It was the end of the trip. I was in our hotel room, working. Anxiety struck when my then eleven-year-old returned from skiing, and I knew something was wrong. As a rule, both sons reflexively announce themselves with a question or bodily function whenever they enter a room. ("Can I watch TV?" "Where's MOM?" Belch.) But . . . silence, until he was in front of me. He'd been crying.

"What's wrong?"

"I lost a glove." More tears.

"That's okay. It's only a glove."

"You don't understand. Mommy just bought me these. They cost eighty pounds. That's a lot of money. She's going to be angry."

"She'll understand. I lose stuff all the time."

"But I don't want her to buy me another pair—they were eighty pounds."

Easy for me to be empathetic. My son's tendency to lose stuff is likely inherited. My ex-wife said if my penis wasn't attached, we'd run across it in Soho on a card table next to a stack of secondhand books and a script for *Goodfellas*. I (no joke) don't carry keys ... what's the point?

So, I got this. We agreed to retrace his steps. Along the way my mind raced: Was this a life lesson? Would buying him a new pair be coddling? I looked down—he was crying. And instantly I was nine years old again.

MUNITIONS

After my folks split, our household income was $800 a month. My mom was always smart and hardworking. Soon our income increased to $900 a month, when she got not one but two raises—the munitions in the battle of me and her against the world. I told Mom, at the age of nine, that I didn't need a babysitter, as I knew we could use the additional $8 a week. Also, my sitter was a religious freak who, when the ice-cream truck came by, gave each of her kids 30 cents and me 15, and who, whenever I said "God," would make me stand in a corner of the living room and hold my arms out, horizontally, like Christ. It really hurt.

"It's Winter; You Need a Jacket"

Said my mom, so off to Sears we went. We bought a size too big, as my mom figured I could go two, maybe three years with this jacket. It cost $33. (This was before fast fashion, which, on an inflation-adjusted basis, may have driven down apparel prices 80 to 90 percent in the past forty years.)

Two weeks later, I left my jacket at my Patrol 42 (Boy Scouts) meeting, but I assured my mom we'd get it back at the next meeting. We didn't.

So off to get another jacket, this time to JCPenney. Mom told me this one was my Christmas present, as we wouldn't have the funds for gifts after buying another jacket. I don't know if this was true or if she was trying to teach me a lesson. Likely both. Regardless, I tried to feign excitement at my early Christmas present, which, incidentally, also cost $33. OPEC is no match for the cartel of outerwear manufacturers and department stores in the 1970s. Sears and JCPenney were so shitty for so long; the real news story is not that they went out of business, but why it took so long.

Several weeks later I . . . lost the jacket. I sat at home after school, in fear, waiting for my mom to come home and absorb another body blow to our already economically enfeebled household. I heard the key turn, she walked in, and I told her:

"I lost the jacket. It's okay, I don't need one . . . I swear."

I felt like crying—bawling, really. However, something worse happened. My mom began to cry. Then she composed herself, walked over to me, made a fist, and pounded on my thigh several times as if she were in a boardroom trying to make a point and my thigh was the table she was slamming her fist on. I don't know if it was more upsetting or awkward. She then went upstairs to her room. She came down an hour later, and we never spoke of it again. Economic anxiety is high blood pressure, and so many Americans know it's always there, waiting to turn a minor ailment into a life-threatening disease. Kids who live in low-income households have higher resting blood pressure than kids who live in wealthy ones.

MEANWHILE, BACK IN THE ALPS

A tall-ish dad and his uni-gloved son had been walking for thirty minutes in eight-degree weather. I had composed myself and attempted to take advantage of my son's weakened state by breaking into song about how things aren't important but relationships are. In the midst of this bad Hallmark Channel scene, my son stopped, then sprinted to a small Christmas tree in front of the Philipp Plein store. The same store where, the day before, his eight-year-old brother had tried to convince his dad to buy him a £250 hoodie with a bedazzled skull on the back. On top of the tree, in place of the star, was one electric-blue boy's glove. A good and somewhat inventive Samaritan had found it and placed it within eyeshot of any boy searching for the vibrant accessory.

My son grabbed the glove, sighed, held it to his chest, and visibly felt a mix of relief and reward. Immediately, I was cast back to being his age, flooded, though I have money now, with the unwelcome nuance of economic anxiety, the recognition I picked up early on that my mom and I weren't like everybody else, that we were the poorest people living in our relatively wealthy neighborhood and it was somehow our fault.

I spent the first fifty years of my life pursuing money and relevance. The money makes me feel less insecure and ticks several instinctive boxes, including the need to provide for my family. Today I'm trying to be more focused on moments of engagement with my boys and strengthening our relationship. Listening, disciplining (bad at this), and trying to make thousands of little investments of affection and patience. Trusting and hoping, that when I'm old, upset, and feeling helpless, I will see my own sons and feel a mix of relief and reward.

chapter 3

HIGHER EDUCATION

THE GANG'S ALL HERE

Most boys need to find their tribe, their posse, a group where they feel they belong. Playing team sports is one way, joining a club another. I wasn't aware how much I'd missed out on male camaraderie until I got to UCLA. Parents raise boys, but so do girls, other boys, women, other men.

At the start of my freshman year, I needed a place to live, preferably close to campus. If this happened, I could move out of my mom's apartment and maybe develop a semblance of a social life that involved women. I was seventeen, a young freshman. In the early eighties, frats had a rep as fun party places—when my dad and I toured Annapolis, *Animal House* was being screened that night for all four hundred midshipmen. That wasn't why I wanted to join one. Fraternities had a certain number of live-in spaces for new pledges—inexpensive housing, basically—and I needed to find someplace I could afford.

During rush week, which is when pledges go to parties and socialize with fraternity members in the hope a match ensues, I rushed five different frats. Sigma Chi was my top choice, as it seemed to be made up exclusively of popular, handsome water polo players. Two days into rush week, a Sigma Chi member took me aside—it wasn't going to happen. I spent that night going up and down fraternity row, asking if any of them offered live-ins. The first yes was from Zeta Beta Tau, or ZBT, the world's first and largest Jewish fraternity, though I didn't know that then.

I hit it off with everyone there and got a bid. ZBT had something called Pledge Pinning, which is Latin for extreme, out-of-control hazing after which the broken-down survivors are awarded some kind of ceremonial trinket. The new pledges, thirty-five of us, showed up at a party, where we were greeted with one hundred bottles of André Cold Duck pink champagne. Our task was to drink three bottles apiece.

Within the hour, half of us were vomiting. One pledge, a guy named Jamie Schwartz, was basically blacked out, his eyes rolling back into his skull. Since I happened to be throwing up on the same couch as Jamie, it's kind of amazing I remember the ensuing conversation as well as I do. *Jamie should go to bed and sleep it off*, someone said. *Maybe we should take him to the ER*, came another voice. The ER idea won. When Jamie got there, he was breathing six times a minute and could have easily died.

That was the first time I got seriously drunk. It put me off alcohol, and so did another drunken night two weeks later when I fell and cracked my head outside our frat house. With the lesson of Jamie still fresh in their minds, the other members hustled me to the ER. The doctor gave me a single stitch in the corner of one eye and sent me home. More traumatizing was the emergency room bill, which came to $320. They asked for an address. Having no money, I had no choice but to forward it to my painfully cheap dad, knowing that when the mail came, he and I would have the ugliest phone call in the world.

My fear was that I'd either have to pay it myself (wasn't sure how) or drop out. But it wasn't so bad. "We got your emergency room bill" was my dad's opening salvo. To his credit, he paid. It wasn't that he didn't have the money—more that he wasn't crazy about spending it on me.

BAND OF BROS

Marriage is great, having children is rewarding, edibles get me to sleep at night, but nothing beats living with a hundred other guys. Despite everything that's been written about them, I'm a hardcore advocate of the Greek system. I get it—frats are responsible for a lot of heinous, ridiculous behavior. Unnecessary injuries and deaths, sexual misconduct, racist incidents, the reckless abuse of alcohol, the list goes on. But if I hadn't joined a frat, it's doubtful I would have lasted long at UCLA. I certainly wouldn't have graduated. Other young men gave me guardrails.

Community, support, acceptance—those were the biggest benefits joining a frat gave me, along with shrinking a university of thirty thousand students down to a manageable size. I'd grown up without having my dad around or any siblings. Suddenly I had a hundred other guys looking out for me while giving me a hard time. Turns out I needed other guys to point out when I was doing well or fucking up. Boys and men can be merciless but, at their best, they provide direction and expectations. I needed that level of socialization, down to a frat brother pushing me to go to campus and chat up and charm a woman and ask if she'd be my date at the upcoming frat formal.

ZBT, like most frats, was close knit. We had no idea how spoiled we were or how good we had it. The other members were mostly wealthy Jewish kids from the Valley. We had a cook who prepared three meals a day—eggs, bacon, and cereal every morning; sandwiches for lunch; a meat loaf or something for dinner—and washed up after us, too. The moms of some of the wealthier boys couldn't get over how awful frat food was, but I found it astonishingly good. Along with being fed and waited on, there was always something new to do—heading over to campus to study or meet women, going out for drinks, staying in, smoking weed, and listening to Pink Floyd. It was like an un-cute Disneyland.

One guardrail came in the form of my Big Brother, Dana Perlman. Every new member got assigned one. In freshman year, Dana told me to quit smoking so much weed. I needed to hear that. In high school, marijuana scared me, but college is about testing and finding your limits, and I'd settled into a twice-weekly stoner's protocol. Dana told me to cut back and make sure I passed all my courses, reminding me I'd already gone to the ER once. Despite his counsel I was placed on academic probation three times. I didn't have enough *good* anxiety yet—it was too easy to dissociate from my responsibilities and enjoy myself (see immature prefrontal cortex). Later, it was the other way around—I suffered too much anxiety, was guilty of too much overthinking, was and still am always thinking the world is about to blow up (see savagely grown-up prefrontal cortex).

Money was still an issue. My dad sent me $200 a month for living expenses, but I was always running out and falling behind. My ZBT roommate also happened to be the frat treasurer—having my bill collector sleeping six feet from me being a huge pain in the ass. By the start of every summer, I regularly found myself $1,000 to $1,500 in the hole, needing to earn twice that much over the next three months for tuition and the first month's house bill in September. *Can you have it by the end of August?* the trustees, always kind, would ask. *Absolutely*, I would answer, knowing if I didn't, I would have to drop out. I lived in the frat all summer, surviving on bananas, Top Ramen, and cereal, and doing every job I could think of, from parking cars to working as a pool boy at the Mondrian Hotel to changing beer taps in bars in Compton and downtown L.A. Meanwhile, my friends were off playing tennis and swimming, traveling to their parents' vacation homes, and interning in their parents' firms.

As time went on, I was elected the president of the UCLA frat council, or basically King of the Jarheads. This involved keeping the three thousand or so men and women within the UCLA Greek system out of serious trouble and coming up with policies and prohibitions around frat parties with blatantly racist and bigoted themes.

DAMN THE TORPEDOES

The death of Tom Petty several years ago hit me as much as any death of a celebrity since Robin Williams. While we don't know celebrities, they can transport us back to a time in our life we usually feel good about. Death is not airbrushed or shot in a soft light, so we see them as more human, empathize, and register our own mortality.

Tom Petty took me back to my freshman year. As a fraternity pledge, I was thrust into a four-man, three-hundred-square-foot room in the fraternity with my "brothers" (total strangers):

- Marty was a big kid from Seattle who had rowed in high school and wore expensive polo shirts. He drove a new Accord and was more ambitious than us at an earlier age. Senior year, he essentially stopped going to class so he could work full-time at a real estate firm. He traded smoking a shit-ton of pot and watching *Planet of the Apes* with friends during the day for the chance to get a nine-month professional jump on us. The rest of us opted to spend sixty, versus sixty-one, years working and experience a year with Charlton Heston, cannabis, and each other. So. Worth. It.
- Pat was from a farm in Visalia. He was also the most creative and likable person any of us had ever met. He was hilarious, outrageous, and fearless, writing songs and scripts and then having us sing and read them, usually very high. Pat and I bonded, as, unlike most of

our brothers, our families were not affluent. We were always broke . . . as in *always*.

- Carl was from the Valley and had a nice innocence about him. He was artistic and constantly doodling, and soon he was designing all the shirts and swag for social events. Claiming it was his psych homework, Pat would put on the theme from *Jaws*, pin another guy named Craig to the ground, and tickle him until he passed out from oxygen deprivation. Then, in the middle of the night, he'd put on the theme from *Jaws* so we could watch Craig wake to the music and reflexively scream "NO!" This still stands as the hardest I've ever laughed.

The soundtrack to all of this in 1983 was Tom Petty's *Damn the Torpedoes* and Bruce Springsteen's *Born in the U.S.A.* albums, which we literally wore out. Hearing of Tom Petty's death inspired a group text around the shock of his passing. I was reminded that Pat had died a decade earlier from what were believed to be complications from AIDS.

Years earlier, at a friend's rehearsal dinner, Pat captivated the table with stories of him being kicked out of his church-sponsored "reeducation" camp—it seems their attempts to turn him straight didn't work. By then, the early 1990s, American society was slowly becoming more accepting of gay people. But at UCLA in the eighties, there was no acceptance whatsoever of gay people or their lifestyle. I couldn't have named a single gay person at UCLA, though several of my good friends, unbeknownst to me, were gay.

So much about who we are and the lives we get to live is a function of where and when we are born, out of our control. I have no choice over my sexuality. Being born a straight man in California in the 1960s was the luckiest stroke that could have happened to me. Being born a gay man in the sixties was the worst thing to happen to Pat.

Born twenty years earlier, Pat could have lived a full adult life. Born ten years later, science would have caught up and made living with HIV manageable.

Most of us have had the chance to do what we dreamed of in college, like finding relevance and achieving a certain level of success. But as you get older, the relationships you have with people you love and who love you overwhelm everything else in your life. It's not something easily explained to a young person. And, unlike most things, we get better at love as we get older. At a minimum, we appreciate it more. Pat was more talented and likable than any of us, but he was robbed of the time to achieve more and have loving relationships wash over those achievements.

When I heard about Tom Petty, I felt sad and nostalgic. I remember Pat and I'm just sad. Very sad.

> **Note:** *As you get older, the relationships you have with people you love and who love you matter more than everything else in your life.*

SOMETHING HAPPENS AT COLLEGE

A recent American theme is that our kids don't need college, that college doesn't matter. This is a blatant lie that parents tell themselves to feel better. It's easier to be named principal dancer at the Kirov Ballet than it is to get a spot in the Ivy League, and then there's the felonious expense of paying for four years of so-called higher education.

College isn't for everyone—but it probably matters as much as it ever has, more even. Find me someone who tells a child, *You don't need college*, and I'll show you a parent who would eat their own legs if their kid got into Harvard.

College is maturity boot camp. I didn't know it then, didn't take my classes seriously, but when I graduated (barely), I was equipped with a more valuable, even marketable skill: the ability to prioritize. I was bombarded by choices and distractions: what classes to take, on which days, taught by which professors; what clubs to join. And then there was friendship, romance, meeting other kids from different backgrounds, calibrating the costs of partying versus staying home and studying—this amounted to a parallel education of arguably more value than what I was nominally there for. I learned to weigh various activities based on their importance and the time they required. Indirectly, I have to believe this leads to improved critical thinking, to knowing "how to think," as the expression goes, even if I never once sat down and took a course with that name.

Romance, sex, and friendship are a few of the defining experiences of college. It's why I'm still so fond of UCLA, despite not learning much, getting mediocre grades, and nearly flunking out. College helped give me an outline. It whittled down and began to clarify and expose who I might be and/or become.

For example, my frat used to host events known as Good and Welfare. At the end of a chapter meeting, members would stand and talk about something, anything. My presentations were always well received. Recognizing I was a good communicator gave me a reputation of sorts. To this day, if there's a skill I could transfer to my kids, it wouldn't be fluent Mandarin or computer programming or even STEM stuff. It would be the tools, the endurance skill, of being a good storyteller. For me, after years of invisibility, it was the beginning of recognizing something I was good at.

> **Note:** *College teaches you critical thinking—how to triage.*

ABOUT FACE, ABOUT MUSCLES

At the end of my freshman year, two other finds finessed my outline: Accutane and rowing crew.

Accutane, a remedy for severe acne, typically takes four to five months to show results, but it took only ten weeks to work on me. My skin was flawless. Not Brad Pitt, but a startling improvement. My body followed. Athletes at UCLA have access to teams of coaches and nutritionists. I was six-two, maybe 160 pounds. After joining the crew team, I was told to add twenty pounds of muscle—four meals and five bananas a day, along with regular weight training. I proceeded to put on a crazy amount of muscle. Between my skin clearing up and my body going from 160 to 180 pounds, I was transformed, to the point of hauling my ass up at five a.m., six days a week, so I could move one-eighth of a shell through the water at speeds supercomputers can't process, only to nearly pass out, throw up from exhaustion, and—wait for it—keep rowing.

These changes paid dividends. I still remember the exact moment a young woman took notice of me. At a frat party, I looked across the crowded room to see Cecilia Barajas. Everyone knew Cecelia—she was Latina, a cheerleader, and beautiful. Our eyes met, I looked away, self-conscious, then looked up again. Cecilia caught my eye. She smiled. It was the first time in my life that an aspirational woman showed any romantic or sexual interest in me.

After losing my virginity—though not to Cecilia—I went a little overboard. Still, it was good for me, a net positive. Everyone goes at his own pace, and my tempo worked for me. One of my most formidable wingmen was my mom. On visits home, if I had a date, she would put logs in the fireplace and leave out a bottle of wine and two glasses. Most parents worry their kids will get into too much trouble—my mom was always worried I wasn't going to get into enough. She basically worked overtime trying to help me get laid. In time, I developed a strong connection with one woman, Margaret, whom I cared a lot about, and who cared for me back. She was and still is wonderful. She and I fell in love. I was with her from the ages of twenty-three to thirty-five, and we later married. Many men never experience a relationship like that—I was extremely fortunate. More about the two of us later.

In college, we all started out as nice, smart, attractive people who had crushes on each other based on a clumsy sense of attraction ("she's hot"/"he's cool"). But by senior year, the women had begun gravitating toward guys who had their shit together, showed early signs of success, or having rich parents, already had the trappings of success, like weekends at their parents' pads in Aspen or Palm Springs.

These women's instincts were kicking in, and they were seeking out mates who could better ensure their offspring's survival—instead of crushing on a funny guy who wore a thin leather tie with Top-Siders and could recite key scenes from the *Planet of the Apes* trilogy.

By senior year, in response, most of my friends were getting their acts together, focusing on grades, grad school, or getting a job. As no good deed goes unpunished, I rewarded the generosity of California taxpayers and the vision of the Regents of the University of California with a 2.27 GPA. I needed a fifth year at UCLA, as I had failed seven classes and didn't have the credits to graduate. Again, not a big deal, as there was more weed and there were more sci-fi movies to be consumed, and nothing compelling waiting for me in the real world.

My senior year, I had a roommate, Gary, who was very ambitious, and I felt an odd sense of competition with him. He was obsessed with becoming an investment banker. I didn't know what investment banking was, but if Gary wanted to do it, I would, too. I interviewed well, lied about my grades—was never called out, either—and was offered a job as an analyst with Morgan Stanley.

My graduation wasn't joyous. It took place midway through my fifth year, with most of my friends gone, as they had done what was expected of them in the standard four years. I spent most of my last two weeks at UCLA asking my professors to change an F to a D so I could get credits for the course and graduate, as I was three courses shy of a BS in economics. I was completely broke. I just had to pass. I had already accepted Morgan Stanley's signing bonus, which was predicated on my graduating. My pitch to the professors was simple and rang true:

I grew up with my mother in a lower-middle-class home.

I have a great job offer from Morgan Stanley in New York.

The sooner I'm out of here, the sooner you can let in someone more deserving.

I asked four profs (there were more I could have asked). Three had the same reaction: they looked at me with disgust, then resignation, signed the form, and asked me to leave their office. No robe and very little pomp and circumstance—more like me sidling away.

LOST, FOUND, LOST

I, too, wanted to increase my selection of mates by signaling resources and success, and Morgan Stanley came to the rescue. I had no idea what investment bankers did, but I understood that being one signaled success.

I fucking hated investment banking. It didn't take me long to realize that the secret is to find something you're good at. The rewards and recognition that stem from being great at something will make you passionate about whatever that something is. Investment banking, for me, was a unique combination of tedious subject matter and lots of stress. Figuring out early that my hunger to impress was leading me down a road of misery gave me the confidence to get out. I quit the path of success devoid of fulfillment, having no idea what I would do instead. I followed the example set by my girlfriend Margaret and my best friend, Adam, and decided to apply to business school. I assumed my bad college grades meant my getting in anywhere was dubious at best, but Adam encouraged me to apply to Berkeley, UCLA, and a bunch of other schools—Duke, Indiana, UPenn, Stanford, Austin, the University of Texas, and Northwestern. One waitlisted me, while the others, bedazzled by my 2.72 GPA, told me to get lost. But California and its taxpayers took another chance on me, and I ended up enrolling in Berkeley's Haas School of Business.

Business schools typically are overflowing with what I call the Elite and the Aimless—mostly smart, accomplished, impressively credentialed kids who know what they don't want to do (whatever their first job out of college was). Most B-schools are a mix of former investment banking analysts like me and former consultants. The ex-consultants all want to go into investment banking, and the ex–investment banking analysts all want to go into consulting. It would be useful, and save time, if someone pointed out accurately that both options are dismal, and suck. Business schools offer optionality, above all else. They increase a graduate's currency in the marketplace. In that way, they're like finishing schools albeit with case studies. I genuinely believe the most talented undergrads can skip business school for the simple reason they don't need it.

AND THEN . . .

In my second year at Berkeley, my mom was diagnosed with an aggressive form of breast cancer. Between smoking her whole life and the birth control pill, which in her day had up to seventeen times the amount of hormones it does now, it wasn't a question of if my mom would get breast cancer but when. Prematurely discharged from Kaiser Permanente hospital in Los Angeles, she started chemo. She called me at Berkeley and said she was feeling awful. I flew home that afternoon and walked through the door into our dark living room. My mom was lying on the couch, in her robe, contorted and vomiting into a trash can, distraught. She looked at me and asked, "What are we going to do?" It rattles me just to write this.

We were underinsured, and I didn't have any contacts who were doctors. I felt a rush of emotions. I wanted to help more than I could, beyond showing up. I wished I had more money and influence, knowing that wealth, among other things, brought contacts and access to a different level of healthcare. We had neither. I felt helpless, angry, and ashamed, as though I'd failed as a son. According to one study, twenty million people (nearly one in twelve adults) in the United States owe medical debt and, of those, approximately fourteen million people, or 6 percent, owe over $1,000. Along with the financial strain, this can't help but take an enormous toll on them emotionally; e.g., *I'm so pathetic I can't even afford to pay for my kid's root canal.*

The following year, I graduated from Berkeley, having gotten my act together (or something) and earned my MBA. I was selected to be the student speaker at commencement and remember looking up, mid-speech, and seeing my mom, cancer marching through her, amid a sea of thousands of parents sitting in the glaring sun at Berkeley's Greek Theatre. She was standing, as she couldn't contain her pride, waving at me with both hands.

I don't believe in an afterlife, but I plan to indulge in a lot of psilocybin before I check out, as I'd like to have some of the bright-light visions people describe when they are near death. I hope I will see two visions: one of my kids rolling on top of my wife and me in bed, laughing, and the image of my mom standing and waving as if she needs to remind me she's there and that she is my mother.

CODA

My childhood, teens, and college years were the stuff of Han Solo, beer, road trips, random sexual encounters, and self-discovery. Pure magic. State-sponsored education is who I am and how I got here. My admittance to UCLA is singular. No other event or action has had a more positive impact on my life and the lives of people around me.

From the mid-twenties on, though, shit starts getting real. The slope of the trajectory for your career is (unfairly) set in the first five years postgraduation. If you want the trajectory to be steep, you'll need to burn a lot of fuel. The world is not yours for the taking but for the trying. The ratio of time you spend sweating to watching others sweat is a forward-looking indicator of your success. Show me a guy who watches ESPN every night, spends all day Sunday watching football, and doesn't work out, and I'll show you a future of rage, menacing silences, and failed relationships. Show me someone who sweats every day and spends as much time playing sports as watching them on TV, and I'll show you a young man who is good at life.

Getting good at life means working.

> **Note:** *The ratio of time you spend sweating to watching others sweat is a forward-looking indicator of your success.*

chapter 4

WORK

Dynasty, Dallas, The Love Boat, and *Fantasy Island* were popular shows when I was in college, which I interpreted as outlining an escape route—through money. And the way I would get money, and develop as a person, was and still is . . . work.

For me, jobs were formative and transformative. The learning curve is basic: when people pay you, they expect you to do your job, or you'll be fired. Work also gave me empathy and social skills and taught me how to handle stressful situations. When I was younger, I'd mostly end up getting fired or I'd quiet-quit. For example, in college I'd be hungover and show up late or be having lunch with a friend and remember suddenly I was due at work two hours earlier. I was talented and a hard worker . . . and then I would say something stupid or make an inappropriate joke and get canned. Things haven't changed much. The jobs I did through college, however, paid enough, along with $5,000 in student loans and Pell Grants, to get me through UCLA with little help from anyone.

My first job was when I was eight or nine, walking a neighbor's dog. I showed up late the first day, blew it off the second, and on the third was—politely—laid off. Later, my mom, underwhelmed by the local pool of babysitters, paid me to babysit myself after school until she came home from work. In my teens, I worked a bunch of jobs (usher, soda and popcorn guy) in various local movie theaters, and as a box boy at Vicente Foods, making $3.50 an hour, or $60 a week, which at the time felt like a shit-ton of money. I did the same in college at Westward Ho, a Brentwood supermarket, along with bagging groceries and lugging them out to people's cars. Rich people were portrayed in the media as grasping and cruel, but I remember thinking how generous and kind they were, noticing that the nicer the car, the friendlier the people, the better the tip.

At Westward Ho, I developed a friendship with a cashier, a single mom, mid-forties, two kids. She was always nice to me, and I liked her, too. She'd been in a terrible car accident, and her mouth and jaw were noticeably deformed. One day, she trailed me into the break room. "I want you to be honest," she said. "Have you noticed my jaw?" We were friends; she was relying on me to tell the truth. This incited in me one of my earliest attempts at kindness. "No," I said, "what are you talking about?" She literally exhaled, her relief was that intense.

This has nothing to do with work—just a reminder to be kind, including in moments when you're called on to show kindness.

My griftiest job involved selling gold coins. It was good training from a sales standpoint but mortifying otherwise. The offices were in Beverly Hills as it sounded tonier on paper or at least less douchey. There was a nice front office in case, you know, anyone got suspicious, but it was basically a ratty, boiler-room operation. No matter the address, there's an underbelly.

A bunch of other broke UCLA students and I were given a list of people to cold-call. When they picked up, I went into the spiel provided by our bosses. Our gold coins were the world's best-performing asset class, with one catch: we were currently sold out. But would they be interested in a future opportunity? If yes, I'd wait seven to ten days, then call again with the electrifying news that our gold coin supply had been replenished and if they were still interested, I'd be willing to set aside three or four. Back at home, I felt like taking a thousand showers to rinse off.

In college, I worked as a pool boy at the Mondrian Hotel. I helped change beer taps in high- and low-end restaurants and bars from Malibu to downtown L.A. Four times a week, I was a sperm donor at a clinic in West L.A., making $640 a month, which basically underwrote my junior year in college. I quit only when my mom pointed out that my biological son might well end up marrying my biological daughter with neither being the wiser. I never checked with the agency—maybe someday.

My first "real" "company" was Stressbuster, a video rental delivery service my friend Lee and I launched in business school. We found a video store with a "Going Out of Business" sign. The stock was a landfill of 1970s and '80s inanity—*Turner & Hooch* and *Fletch* and *Can't Stop the Music*—along with some decent films like *Hannah and Her Sisters* and *Witness*. Videos that went for $23 new were being sold for $3 apiece—we later learned the store had been busted by the FBI for money-laundering. Pooling our money, Lee and I bought four hundred videos and stored them in my mom's storage locker in our apartment building garage. Then we drove over to the Twin Towers in Century City, bribed the security guards, and went from floor to floor, trying to convince people to rent *The Swarm*.

It was tiring, humiliating work. Some people were friendly, others surly. I was kicked out of many offices. *Get out! Get out!* one woman shouted at me, which shook me so much I slammed the office door on my fingers. *This whole thing sucks*, I thought. A week or so later, when I went to retrieve the videos from my mom's storage locker, it was empty—ransacked. Like a good neighbor, State Farm Insurance, of all things, ended up buying us out for $2,500. I remember proudly telling my B-school classmates my business had been "acquired" by State Farm.

CliffsNotes: Low-paying jobs, particularly first jobs, are generally shitty. That is as it should be—almost everybody with a great job now started out doing something tedious and difficult for not much money. How do you make a lot of money? Answer: by starting to make money... any money. I was once paid $18 an hour to count the number of cars that entered and exited a parking lot. One cashier lit into me for overstuffing a grocery bag, while another was Ms. Congeniality. Working teaches you about other people. You gain empathy and compassion. You begin to recognize and own your skills. You do the quiet math: If I smile and am friendly to people, I'll get a tip. If I keep the ice bucket full, the bartenders will remember me later in cash. If I don't get stoned tonight, I'll be less mentally obtuse at work in the morning. I learned about labor unions, and substance abuse on the job, how many people depend on drugs and alcohol to sand the edges of their workday. When you're a white frat boy at UCLA, doing these jobs gives you a kaleidoscopic glimpse of what feels like the real world.

It's why, for young people, an early job is as much about socialization as it is about cash. You learn how to work on a team, how to deal with coworkers and managers and customers, who can be jerks. You learn how to persuade and how to get people to buy something from you and how to survive in a capitalist economy. In sum, you start to learn that if you want success, you have to work for it—and that often means being willing to sacrifice for it. Few things build a young person's self-respect, sense of purpose, and willingness to buy into society more than their first paycheck. Finally, working these jobs hardened me to rejection and hearing "No." I learned to be scrappy and resilient.

TO SERVE AND PROTECT

I'm a big believer that a young man should have at least one experience in the service industry. This summer, I'm making my oldest son, Alec, work as a waiter/dishwasher in a burger restaurant—he'll learn a ton. Service work is boot camp, elemental training for life. You learn things you don't even realize you're being taught. Today, I'm just

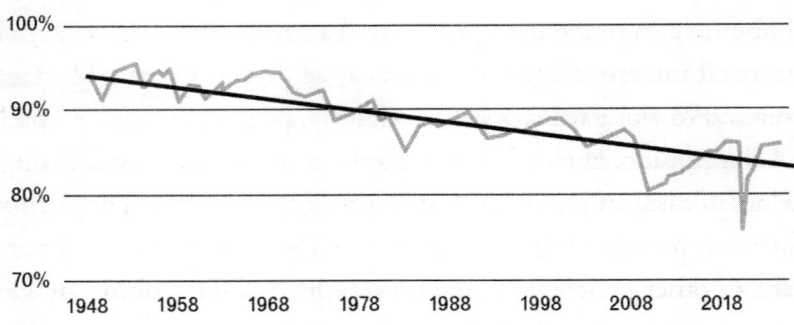

a mild asshole—hard to imagine how awful I'd be if I hadn't worked service jobs, in my case half a dozen or so.

First, working in a restaurant, fast-food outlet, or retail store requires a baseline of mental fortitude to propel you to get out of bed on an overcast morning, change into a uniform, and show up at work on time. Waiting tables, busing plates and bowls, serving drinks, and bagging groceries is a form of athleticism. You're running back, forth, up, and down, managing responsibilities in a tense, clamorous environment that's always changing. Someone's lunch is late or cold or they need a drink refill, the fryer is smoking, the card reader is frozen—and you have to deal with it. Service industries also create incentives via real-time compensation, usually tips in exchange for speed, proficiency, and good manners. That's much better training for life than sitting at a desk, analyzing a spreadsheet.

Every service job I worked, whether I liked or hated it, turned into a blessing. Service jobs are the Diet Coke version of national service. As a kid, I had no idea I lacked empathy, but working a job where you deal with the public teaches you you're no different from the people on the other side of the counter. They have the same hopes and dreams as you do. It's virtually impossible to be an asshole if you're a bartender or waiter. You'll get nowhere if you scream at and curse out your coworkers or are selfish or incompetent at what you do. You can't help leave these jobs a kinder, more patient, altogether better person.

You help improve the world, too. You begin to appreciate your own good fortune relative to others. If you grew up privileged and never had to work at Burger King or Subway or Marshalls or Chick-fil-A, it's not inconceivable you'll grow up seeing the world through the lens of caste and think everyone is here to serve you. They're not. A key component of great leadership is the ability to walk, figuratively, in other people's shoes. Service jobs disabuse you of the idea you're an exception to the rule.

They also provide much-needed immunity against the notion of American meritocracy. I once worked as a dishwasher in a fast-food hamburger joint. My coworkers, mostly Mexican and Central American immigrants, all worked their asses off for minimum wage. At night, after the place closed, they plugged in a small, ancient black-and-white TV and a VCR, snapped open a six-pack of Budweiser, and sat around watching porn—their treat at the end of a hectic day. I was applying to UCLA at the time, feeling sorry for myself that I couldn't afford some of what my classmates could. Seeing my coworkers drinking Bud and watching grainy sex scenes while acknowledging what little money they were making helped me appreciate what I had.

In the United States, the concept of meritocracy has a dark side. If you don't end up working at Goldman Sachs and living in Brooklyn Heights and socializing at the hottest clubs, the message is plain: *You screwed up—it's your fault.* Such bullshit. My coworkers saved money by living together in small quarters and sent most of their paychecks home to their families in Mexico, Honduras, Guatemala, and El Salvador. They worked harder than me and spoke better English. But I was born a white, straight man in Laguna Niguel, California. I realized: life in the United States isn't a meritocracy or even close. Yes, individuals have agency—but some individuals have more than others. Service work is an anti-meritocracy vaccine, a reminder that the

American Dream for some people is closer to a hallucination, given how many people sleep with one eye open, worrying about how they're going to pay for their kid's asthma medication.

Finally, service jobs are early training for delivering surplus value. Anyone under the age of eighteen has negative value. They take in much more than they give. Now, suddenly, they're in a workplace situation where they have to fetch someone's Prius, serve half a dozen lunches, and ring up strangers. It instills humility. It activates the mirror neurons. For young men especially, it's a rehearsal for learning how to be in the service of others.

> **Note:** *Every young man should work a service job at least once. It's a vaccine against the idea of meritocracy. You also gain empathy.*

REAL WORLD, REAL JOB

I accepted Morgan Stanley's analyst offer because (a) I was extremely economically motivated, and (b) rumor had it Morgan Stanley didn't bother to check college transcripts or drug-test its applicants and employees. I lied about my grades and was lucky to be interviewed by a guy who rowed crew in college. "Oarsmen get an automatic offer, as you're willing to kill yourself in pursuit of a goal," he said. Okay, then. My first day, I was asked to pee in a jar, but I assumed the company was on the lookout for coke and meth, not weed, because no one followed up.

I hated investment banking, I was terrible at it, too, but the two years I spent there had value. The eighty-nine other analysts in my class were far more skilled, disciplined, and academically credentialed than me, which made me (generously) the company's eighty-eighth best analyst. (My fault: UCLA is a sink-or-swim place; I decided to do neither and smoke pot and tread water.) Analyst #89 was (no joke) escorted out of 1251 Avenue of the Americas by the FBI and convicted of insider trading.

Most jobs are either high-stress and rewarding or low-stress and boring. An ER doctor's life is stressful but also variable and interesting (at least on *ER*, *Gray's Anatomy*, and *The Pitt*). Guarding museum paintings is low-stress but, I'm guessing, tedious as shit. Investment banking is unique in that it combines boring, arid material with air traffic controller levels of screaming stress. The jobs people are paid top dollar for generally fall into this category of boring and nerve-wracking. Being a partner in a niche law firm is benumbing and pressure filled; it also pays crazily well. At Morgan Stanley, right out of UCLA, I was making more money than any of my friends, but what I was actually doing was going back and forth to the printer every night until four a.m. and proofing and printing prospectuses for municipal bond offerings. Was it the base rental *payment* or *payments* with an s? One tiny error in an eighty-page prospectus and I'd get fired. The other analysts and I had to show up in the morning before the senior execs, most of whom also hated their jobs but were imprisoned by their high salaries and "lifestyles," and we couldn't leave until they left, no matter how late it got. There was lots of yelling. A VP once threw a chair at me. The culture was stupid, abusive, racist, and sexist. I loathed it.

Morgan Stanley has gotten significantly better since, but the culture back then was decidedly unhealthy. The lowest-paying jobs, including mailroom employees, were held by Black employees, which served to promote unconscious or, if you like, flagrant racism. There were no female associates, VPs, or managing directors. One of the few women analysts in our group was fired halfway through the program. I'm pretty sure if I'd committed whatever offense she had, I would have kept my job—after all, my boss and I used to attend UCLA games together. Most of the top jobs were filled by white men who'd gone to really good schools. Worst was the conflation of talent and awful behavior. If you were a nice guy and a talented analyst, good going, boss.

But talented *and* an asshole meant you were . . . legend. The guy who threw the chair at me? Mythical, plus anyone that passionate had to be a baller at his job.

However, I'm glad I did it. I developed focus, excellent reading skills, and an attentiveness to detail that's served me well my whole life. The job also showed me what I *didn't* want. I would show up at the office on Tuesday morning at nine a.m. and leave the next day at five p.m. Working thirty-two hours straight became a routine. The company culture encouraged a muscular mono-focus. Whenever analysts pulled an all-nighter, they would be awarded a clean white shirt. By the end of the year, I had the most white shirts of anyone there, which is either good or depressing.

Crew was excellent prep. There comes a point in every rowing race, at around eight hundred meters, when your body starts giving out. Your legs are so exhausted you can't feel them. The air passing through your esophagus is a tiki torch. There are twelve hundred meters to go, and unless you play mental tricks, you'll pass out. That point, when you think you can't go on a second longer, means you're at 40 percent of your actual limit. Humans are remarkable that way. Most of us never reach 40 percent, much less 100 percent, of our capabilities. We tell ourselves we're testing our outermost limits when we're not even close, the result being we're never called on to develop real resilience and courage. Working thirty-two hours straight was easy—doctors and medical residents do it all the time. All I needed was a couch, a short nap, and coffee, and I rolled back to my desk.

Though I hated investment banking, I loved making money, and I was in a wonderful, loving relationship, too. (I was still together with my girlfriend Margaret from college, who worked at Arthur Andersen.) The Morgan Stanley job enabled the two of us to buy a home in Potrero Hill in San Francisco for $285,000 at the age of twenty-eight. Imagine any young person being able (today) to get through college and buy a home in San Francisco with their own earnings. Wouldn't happen.

The United States today doesn't have a housing crisis; it has an affordability crisis. Roughly one-third of Americans rent, and nearly half are "cost-burdened," meaning that they spend 30 percent or more of their income on housing. Since 2019, rents have increased 1.5 times faster than income in most U.S. metro areas. In purely economic terms, increased housing costs reduce labor mobility and productivity, as workers can't afford to live in high-growth areas. When human capital can't be invested in the regions offering the greatest returns, it dampens growth; one research project estimates that removing housing constraints (i.e., lowering costs) to increase the liquidity of human capital would increase GDP by $1.4 trillion. In sum, there may be an economic as well as a social justification for government investments in housing.

Elevated housing costs also take a toll on health, as families who struggle to afford housing often delay medical care, are less likely to be able to afford healthier food, and have higher levels of anxiety and depression. But the most catastrophic consequence of unaffordable housing is that 770,000 Americans experience homelessness. According to one study, communities where the median rent is more than 32 percent of the median household income are likely to see sharply higher rates of homelessness. But no matter where they live, homeless people suffer intense physical and mental harm, put a

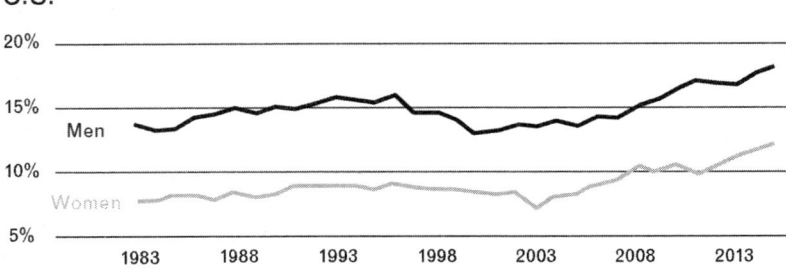

Percentage of 25- to 30-Year-Olds Living in Parental Home
U.S.

Source: U.S. Census, DB Global Markets Research.

disproportionate burden on public services, and reduce the quality of life for all citizens.

The common denominator for struggling renters and the homeless? It isn't any type of identity but money. Increasing support for Section 8 housing and rent control may provide short-term relief, but in the long term these programs become entrenched and suppress development. The quickest way to help poor people afford housing is simple: pay them more. The minimum wage should be $25 an hour.

At the end of my second year, I had to decide: Should I try to do a third year, possibly make the jump up to Morgan Stanley associate? It didn't matter if investment banking wasn't for me: it was work—and money. My body said no.

I woke up one day to a weird fluttering in my chest. Maybe I'd swallowed a bird. I went to the doctor, who did a heart test, diagnosed me with ventricular tachycardia, or an abnormal heart rhythm, and ordered me hospitalized. Two weeks earlier, the top college basketball player in the country, Hank Gathers, had just completed a monster slam dunk and was running back up the court when he fell to the floor and unfortunately died. V-tach was in the news.

I ended up at the ICU of Saint John's Hospital in Santa Monica. I

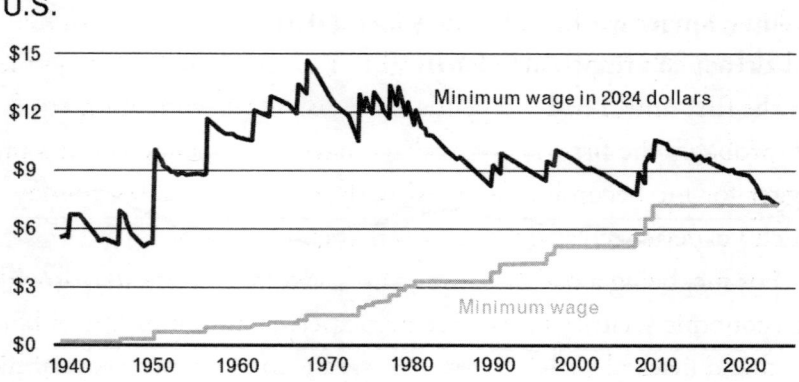

Federal Minimum Wage
U.S.

Source: Bureau of Labor Statistics.

was twenty-four years old and surrounded by elderly people recovering from quadruple-bypass surgeries. A social worker came by. "Why are you here?" she asked. When I began explaining, she said, "No, no, no. I mean, why are you here?" I had no answer. Then and there, I decided to leave investment banking.

> **Note:** *Your body will sometimes make decisions for you when your brain won't. Learn to listen to your body.*

SOME NOTES ON WORK

For thirty-five years, most of my waking hours, effort, skills, and even relationships have been focused on work. Is that dysfunctional, or American? The answer is yes. While my wife and two boys mean more to me now, work has constituted my identity and was the greatest source of reward for so long.

Initially my focus on work was driven by wanting to impress women—including my mom—and gaining access to a broader selection of mates. Capitalism creates an operating system where the incentives to make money are irresistibly strong. Today, America is more itself than ever: a loving, generous place if you have money, and a rapacious, violent one if you don't.

My focus on work turned serious when my mom got sick. She could no longer work, and I knew I would need to take care of her. I had already felt responsible for her, but now she relied solely on me. For the first time, I had a dependent—it was a real-world moment for me, probably the first. I soon realized having a dependent was a big trigger for me becoming obsessed with work and making money—which I experienced again when my first child was born.

For me, being a dad at first meant . . . work. Specifically, providing economic security for the science experiment brandishing a blue wristband marked with my surname. Sadly, the first two years of his life, I was barely there. Same with his younger brother. While their mom, my wife, needed my support, I had found no evidence that babies yearned for their dad (can't wait for the hate on this), but I felt an almost catatonia-inducing amount of pressure to provide for their future. Yes, they recognized me and smiled . . . as they did with the dog, nanny, mobile, and toaster oven. (Maybe I was under my dad's spell initially.) But I felt the utter responsibility of bringing new life into this world and so I turned to work. (Keep reading, as this conflicts with my main parenting advice later.)

I'm not alone in looking back on a life defined by work. It has defined the modern age, conveniently. Our work constitutes our economy, it occupies most of our time, and it often can determine our friendships, mates, geography, and health and welfare. English is supposed to be the most nuanced language, with more words to provide more texture to communicate. Yet it falls short on the word "work," as the concept covers a surface area that the single syllable can't encapsulate.

DON'T FOLLOW YOUR PASSION

Show up at any high school or college commencement ceremony, and the guest speaker will regale you with yeasty bromides. Follow your passion. Do what you love, and the rest will take care of itself.

Here's some counter-advice: Don't. Rather, those few people who can, and make a serious living at it, are highly unusual and lucky. Yup, I add my name to this category. I never dreamed of starting a brand strategy firm, then analytics, then e-commerce—I would have much rather been the starting QB for the New York Jets or a French heartthrob. Nor at any point in my career as a strategy consultant did I think, *Living the dream!* It was more that I was pretty good at it, the work was both interesting and difficult, the market seemed willing to pay me and my firm to keep doing it, and maybe economic security would follow.

I don't mean to crush people's passions. If you're dead set on being a jewelry designer or an opera singer, give it your best shot. But unless there are economic rewards, it's not enough to be great at something. Consider implementing metrics: if you're not doing/haven't accomplished X or Y by the age of X or Y, you might think about a profession that's more economically viable. Regardless, you still need to be super-lucky, as evidenced by the fact that a disproportionate percentage of the people who succeed in glamour jobs are nepo babies.

Instead of passion, identify what you're good at and focus on it. Find something you could, in time, be great at, that has a 90+ percent employment rate, and that the internet can't easily shred or supplant. Making money may not be top of mind when you'd rather be out drinking cold ones, but later it will, when even the most quixotic unemployed Broadway actor allergic to the normies will admit the value of having a good day job.

Does it sound like I'm advocating selling out; i.e., finding a well-paying but unrewarding desk job? No—all I'm saying is that becoming good, or great, at candle-making or installing soapstone countertops, and the pride you'll feel, along with the economic accoutrements, and the camaraderie and praise you get, can help clarify and deepen that passion. Talk to someone who makes a great living as a family dentist or as the CEO of a paper and packaging supply company, and I'll show you someone who's kind of interested in periodontal disease and/or corrugated cardboard. As you get older, what drives passion changes. You get passionate about taking care of your kids, taking your partner on a great vacation, picking up the check for the whole table. Not saying you can't be happy without money, just that it makes life a whole lot easier.

My passion? I think I'm a decent communicator. At UCLA, I was known as a really good orator. I remember thinking, *How can I make money speaking?* At a UCLA career fair, one or two people told me I should become a corporate spokesperson. No idea what that was. I was, I also realized, a good teacher. Public speaking, writing, and consulting (i.e., conveying business ideas to a group or board) followed. Still, the difference today between me and a lot of the people you see on the speaking circuit is that I have an ability to attract and retain really talented people who can turn my rubbing alcohol into rocket fuel.

Along with focusing on what you're good at, the strongest indicator of future success is your perseverance and resilience. Unless you are supremely disciplined, your career will have to be something that gives you some enjoyment. But don't mistake focus for your "passion." Follow your talent. Put yourself in a position to be financially successful. Get certified: in a digital world, much of the corporate world decides whether to swipe right or left based on the logos (aspirational universities and firms, vocational certifications, etc.) on your LinkedIn page.

Again, money matters. As someone who grew up without much of it, I know how its absence can be a colossal stressor. It's a preservative of good health, attendant longevity, and the happiness that comes from taking care of your spouse and children. I learned this early on, after my dad left and we went from living in a fairly nice house to living in a fairly crappy apartment, and I began attending a high school with metal detectors. When you're a kid, you'll have fun regardless of where you live, but I immediately sensed the strain on my mom. *She's divorced and upset*, I thought. Then I realized her biggest source of stress was that we didn't have enough money, that when she freaked out if the vacuum cleaner broke, it was because we didn't have the money to get it fixed. Quite frankly, one reason I may be more economically successful than some of my friends is that I was motivated never to have to be in those circumstances again. Few things make me crazier than hearing a venture capitalist claiming their success was never about money, that they just wanted to build something great and the money followed. Having advised a lot of these types, I know for a fact they can tell you that minute and hour how much they're worth.

Money is also a luxury that allows you to think about and do other things. Everyone has a fulcrum—mine was working nonstop for thirty years so I could hit, then exceed, my economic goal. That was my way; I'm not saying it's the right way. Other people don't live to work; they work to live. They move to a lower-cost city or town; have a good job and a partner who may or may not work; prioritize their kids, family, church, community, hobbies, and/or giving back. They live really good lives. In America this is getting harder to do, because (a) the number of people who can lead an adequate life here has declined dramatically because of the costs of real estate, healthcare, education, and food; (b) the pressure, temptation, and rewards of having money have never been greater; and (c) it's kind of unbelievable what money can buy.

These days I'm spending more time with people and projects I care about, at the expense of earning money, because I can afford to. Not sure I would have been able to balance the stress of not being economically comfortable with prioritizing relationships and family when I was younger. I do now. I'm working at being more in the moment and turning down certain economic opportunities so I can do more stuff focused on the condition of my soul, if it's not too late. Anyone can do this at any time, by the way, money or no money.

> **Note:** *Don't follow your passion professionally. Find what you're good at—and follow your talent. The rewards and recognition that stem from being great at something will make you passionate about that something.*

STAY HUNGRY

I think a lot about success and its underpinnings. Talent is key, but it will only gain you entrance to a crowded VIP room. Kind of like Platinum Medallion on Delta—you think you're special, but at LaGuardia, you realize there are a lot of you. Let's assume you are exceptionally talented. Maybe even in the top 1 percent. Congrats: you join 75 million people, the population of Germany, all vying for more than their share of the world's resources.

The chaser that takes talent over the top and into success is hunger. Hunger can come from a lot of places. I don't think I was born with it. I have a great deal of insecurity and fear, which, coupled with the instincts we all have and probably some of what I went through as a kid, has resulted in hunger. Ambition isn't always pretty. Understanding where hunger comes from can illuminate the difference between success and fulfillment.

> **Note:** *Talent isn't enough. Being in the 1 percent means joining 75 million others.*

Rx: CONFUSION

If you're in your twenties, forgive yourself if you're clueless about what you'll do professionally and/or with the rest of your life. Some kids know early on—they're freakishly proficient at one thing—but odds are you're not one of them. I wasn't. In a confused, auditioning state is where you should be—not adrift, but sorting out options. At age nine, I thought I was going to be a baseball pitcher. I found out that wasn't going to happen when I hit adolescence. Then I wanted to be a pediatrician. Chemistry disabused me of that notion. Then I was going to become an investment banker. I sucked at it. In business school I decided I would work for a healthcare consultancy, but instead I became an entrepreneur and started a company, Prophet, then sold it, then started another company, followed by seven more, two home runs, the others bunts, infield flies, and a strikeout.

The key is not to waste away in your confusion. Instead let it light up your curiosity.

If you're in business school, it already means you don't know what you'll do. At Haas, I had no vision—I didn't even think about having one. Most students know only that they don't want to be doing what they're doing at that moment. They're hoping to pivot, using business school as a lever to get them elsewhere, ideally for more money. B-school is like rehab minus the alcohol and drugs, with great nutrition and weights, the promise being that you'll emerge better, stronger, and more attractive to the marketplace.

On my B-school application, I wrote that I wanted to start an information systems software company. I didn't know what information systems were, still don't. If you're smart, your goal in your twenties is to be workshopping, talking to people, trying things out. Be thoughtful... Any opportunity you have when you're young to choose among different paths is a profound blessing. Along the way, you're investing in relationships and platforms—high school and college alumni networks, industry get-togethers, your own organization—that increase your viability in the workplace. Talk to other people. Heed their assessments of where you are, ignore some of it, take the rest to heart. How can you tell the difference? If friends and colleagues are being mean, or vindictive, feel free to discount it. But if what they say feels like a gut punch, if it causes you to pause and think, *Shit*, it's likely true.

In my online teacher reviews at NYU, I get some variations of "Scott's an asshole" or "Scott's a dick." That's plenty fair. Several times, though, students comment that my profanity and self-absorption reduce my credibility—that I seem more focused on myself than on the subject material. Every time this comes up, I get rattled. Why? Because it's true. If an outside assessment throws you off balance, feels like you've just been told really bad news, it's usually a telltale sign.

> **Note:** *Your goal in your twenties is to be workshopping, talking to people, trying out new things. Be thoughtful... Any opportunity you have when you're young to choose among different paths is a blessing.*

My life has always been in, around, or adjacent to technology. I could have easily ended up working in energy, but I graduated from Berkeley in the thick of the 1990s tech boom. Plan all you want, but the random opportunism of life often derails those plans or sparks new ones.

After B-school, I immediately got offers from consulting firms. What tiny bits of self-awareness I had reminded me that I lacked the skills to be an effective employee inside a big company. I'd be an entrepreneur instead.

> **Note:** *Almost no one has a career map. Put one foot in front of the other and see where it takes you.*

BORING IS SEXY

Careers are asset classes. If a sector becomes overinvested with human capital, the returns on those efforts, in general, are suppressed (note: Morgan Stanley and financial services tend to be exceptions to this). If you want to work at *Vogue*, produce movies, or open a *crêperie*, you need to ensure that you receive a great deal of psychic income, as the returns on your efforts (apart from well-publicized exceptions) will be, on a risk-adjusted basis, awful. I try to avoid investing in anything that sounds halfway cool. I didn't buy *BlackBook* magazine or invest in a downtown members-only club focused on dubcore. If, on the other hand, the business, and the issue it addresses, sound so boring I want to jump out the window, then . . . bingo, I'll invest. A few years ago, I spoke at the J.P. Morgan Alternative Investment Summit, where the bank hosts three hundred of the wealthiest families in the world. There are some who own media properties or a national airline, but most killed it in smelting, insurance, or pesticides.

AFTER GRADUATION . . .

For the first twenty-four to thirty-six months after graduation, young men are advised to embrace a degree of stoicism. I enjoy alcohol and THC and used them every day in college. But I took twenty-four months (mostly) off both immediately after graduation as I knew I needed to be in great shape physically and mentally to succeed. Whether shopping, gaming, swiping, posting, eating, looking at porn, streaming, gambling, or watching ESPN, take as much of this energy and time for the next couple years and reallocate that human capital to three areas: work, relationships, and fitness. This focus will pay dividends.

It's monotonous and likely not sustainable. However, the DNA of your career and professional trajectory is disproportionately, unfairly set by the early years of it. Some people bloom in their forties. Most successful people, however, burn a great deal of fuel in their twenties and thirties to ascend through a resistant inner space and make the jump to light speed. They cover greater ground in their forties and fifties thanks to the velocity established in their first twenty professional years.

If you're in your twenties, be mentally and physically a warrior. Lift heavy weights and run long distances, in the gym and in your brain. Many tasks you'll be asked to perform early in your career will be staggeringly boring. Who cares? Don't do only what you are asked to do, but also what you are capable of doing. Embrace the challenge. Think of it as boot camp before being sent to battle, as there are millions of other warriors fighting to win the same regions of prosperity. Get strong, really strong, physically and mentally. The goal is to walk into a room and believe you can vanquish, outrun, or outlast every person in it.

Send a message to your colleagues that you came to play. Many of you will have a gag reflex at my boomer capitalist mentality or some such bullshit. No, it's America—a platform to deploy skills and grit to add value and accumulate resources.

Note: *If you're in your twenties, be mentally and physically a warrior.*

ALL? NOTHING AT ALL?

I was at a conference once when someone asked me about my management philosophy. This was when I was running L2. Everyone wanted to hear about balance and modeling good behavior and befriending your inner child. Mine could be summed up as "I'm all fucking over everybody all the fucking time." The audience gasped. More politely, for me it wasn't about balance—it was about building something great and creating economic security for myself someday.

What of "balance"? Fine—many people thoughtfully calibrate the trade-off and fashion a good life for themselves and their families without being obsessed with work and money. But if you want money, influence, and relevance, assume you are not that person. Make your first act count, have it mean something. Outside of work, I barely remember my twenties and thirties. Work cost me my hair, probably, my first marriage, and arguably my sanity. But for me, it was worth it. I found it's what's required if you expect to be in the top 10 percent economically, much less the top 1 percent.

Balance is a myth. There are only trade-offs. Having balance at my age is a function of lacking it in my twenties and thirties. That's just me. You may feel differently—tens of millions of people do, and they're (no doubt) happier and, well, more balanced than me. Your call. If you prioritize things besides money, recognize this also means making certain compromises; e.g., not living in New York or San Francisco or London, owning a less nice car, traveling only occasionally, waiting in longer lines at Disneyland. A lot of young people tell me they want "balance" while also expecting to make significant money and have influence. When you look at their Pinterest boards, you find dozens of Rolex watches and yearning, late-afternoon photos of the ducks on Georgica Pond. They're not being realistic. Have an honest conversation with yourself about what you want in life and what sacrifices you're willing to make to attain it.

Until my Berkeley graduation, I'd done a reasonably good job with scant commitment. I knew, though, that things would be different moving forward. Soon I would need to take care of a sick parent and demonstrate a level of grit commensurate with the opportunities presented to me. At that moment I felt a sense of accomplishment, that I was loved, but also immense stress that hasn't waned for over three decades. The most rewarding things in life—relationships, work, kids—are all really fucking stressful.

> **Note:** *There's no such thing as balance, only trade-offs. You can have it all, just not at the same time.*

REALITY TEST

As a young man, I thought my success was solely a function of my being awesome. My character, my tenacity, my talent. What a fucking child.

I've built companies, had some success in different forms of media, and am a good (not great) professor. The fire that drove my success was a fear of being broke (again) and desperately needing to feel relevant—to impress my mom and my friends, and to punch above my weight class with women. Again, that's just me. When something really wonderful happens these days, it feels as if it didn't really happen, as I can't call my mom to share the achievement. For more than two decades, she hasn't been there. I'm a sixty-year-old man who still hasn't gotten over the loss of his mother. And that's okay. Truth is, I hope my boys feel some of the same emotions about me when I'm gone. But that's not what this is about.

If I'm generous with myself, I have one skill I'm particularly proud of. I foster a decent amount of loyalty among the people I work with. It's not a function of character or empathy, only the recognition that nothing wonderful happens when you're on an island. It bears repeating: greatness and happiness are in the agency of others. If you aren't willing to engage with coworkers, you won't ever become an effective leader. Corporate America has invented a term for people who are talented but don't want to engage: "sole contributors." This is business Latin for "assholes": people who's talented enough to recognize they can be an asshole (not engage) and still be tolerated. Big tech and media have conflated talent with being a shitty person. No, the two are not correlated—it's that some talented and fortunate people find currency in being an asshole. Most people don't have that luxury. There's a real dignity and grace to people who are super talented and super nice. These are the people who, near the end, get to drop the mic.

> **Note:** *Greatness and happiness are in the agency of others.*

A few other ideas for how to approach work to add surplus value:

GET THE EASY STUFF RIGHT

I've struggled my whole career with this. I used to rally a team to pull together an insightful, hard-hitting presentation and then show up to that presentation fifteen minutes late, pissing everyone off. After the meeting, I'd get an email from the client about additional work or some other opportunity, then not respond in a timely fashion and lose momentum. I was bad at following up with people when I should have done so—and wanted to. In general, a lack of professionalism and bad manners has probably reduced the slope of my trajectory.

The lesson here is easy: don't be the fucking idiot I once was—get the easy stuff right. Show up early. Have good manners. Follow up. Answer the email.

> **Note:** *Get the easy stuff right.*

BELIEVE YOU DESERVE IT

With increased attention and recognition, a guy appears on my shoulder, whispering in my ear, *Who are you kidding? You're a fraud.* I thought that whenever success came my way, it was because I was "fooling" people. I didn't warrant recognition as an academic or rewards as an entrepreneur. I felt an anxiety, always, that I'd be found out for what I really was: the son of a secretary; a person who got mediocre grades in school, did not invest in relationships, was selfish, and wasn't that gifted. Someone whose only real talent was self-promotion and taking credit for other people's work. A fraud.

Seventy percent of Americans admit to experiencing imposter syndrome at least once in their lifetime. That's a lot. Unless you take time to address these thoughts, they get louder, psychologists say. So I cut myself some slack, as I've also worked hard, taken risks, and given back along the way.

Still, that voice is almost always in my ear—*I know who you really are*. I know, but I also hope this insecurity can someday transform into feeling good about who I really am.

KNOW YOUR WORTH

The wind of our society's obsession with big tech is still at my back, running over my vocal cords. These skills, coupled with proprietary data that the Prof G staff collects and distills into insight, and a world-class creative team that designs imagery and charts, shot on the screen behind me, all sing like Pavarotti.

But my market value, like all things, will fade. People will tire of my topics and/or me, and I won't have access to the resources that make my stuff great, versus just good. Or, more likely, my creative juices will just stop flowing. Working with young, creative people and having access to the best and brightest thinkers in business is for me what heroin was to Keith Richards. Once it's gone, no more hits.

My relationship with NYU's Stern School, generally speaking, is that I teach a mess of kids and speak at events. In exchange, they put up with me. Every three or four years a new department chair or administrator asks me to teach more, changes my status, or does something to piss me off. I threaten to go to Wharton or Cornell Tech, and I mostly get what I want. If I sound like a diva or a pain in the ass, trust your instincts. I don't act like an employee at Stern but a free agent, and it frustrates them. My star is still burning bright—I'm good at teaching and I strengthen the Stern brand, so they tolerate me. But when my value begins to wane (and it's only a matter of time), they'll drop me like second-period French.

LEAVE YOUR HOUSE

You should strive never to be at home. Home is for seven hours of sleep and recharging your tech, that's it. The amount of time you spend at home is inversely correlated to your success, professionally and romantically. Get out there not just to meet your colleagues, but also to chat up women, to expand your friend and network groups by interacting with people with different interests, goals, and hobbies, and to develop and refine your own visibility. Along with snatching three-plus years out of everyone's life, Covid created (or validated) isolationist habits. The aftereffects—distrust, distance, paranoia—are with us still. See if you can overcome them.

> **Note:** *The amount of time you spend at home is inversely correlated to your success, professionally and romantically.*

LONE WOLF HOWLING

People romanticize entrepreneurs. But for most, entrepreneurship is a function of the absence of certain abilities. Whether they own a car wash or are trying to launch the next big thing, most entrepreneurs lack either the access or the capacity to enter and survive the greatest wealth-creating vehicle in history, the American corporation.

Do you have access to Google, Salesforce, McKinsey, SpaceX? If so, then fuck being an entrepreneur and take the damn job. On a risk-adjusted basis, if you have the skills, emotional maturity, and tolerance for injustice when someone notably less talented than you gets promoted and you don't, or your email and everyone else's has been turned off overnight with no explanation, or if you can walk into a room without assuming everyone is talking shit about you privately, then do it. (At Morgan Stanley, I lacked these skills.)

Working for a corporation is a great way to get rich slowly. The firm invests resources trying to make you better, and on health insurance so you can get that mole removed. Otherwise, most new businesses meander along or fail. Starting or working for one is a risky, fraught way to make a living. But I've never been afraid to sell and I've always taken risks. "Entrepreneur" is just a synonym for "salesperson," as you're constantly trying to persuade investors, clients, employees, or whomever else it might be.

When students show up at my office hours at NYU, it's almost never to talk about class material or homework. They want job advice. The conversation typically goes like this: *I just got an offer from Fidelity, but I want to start my own business.* My response: *Don't be an idiot, take the job at Fidelity.*

I didn't take my own advice. At B-school, I called all the consulting firms who'd offered me jobs and turned them down. I would start

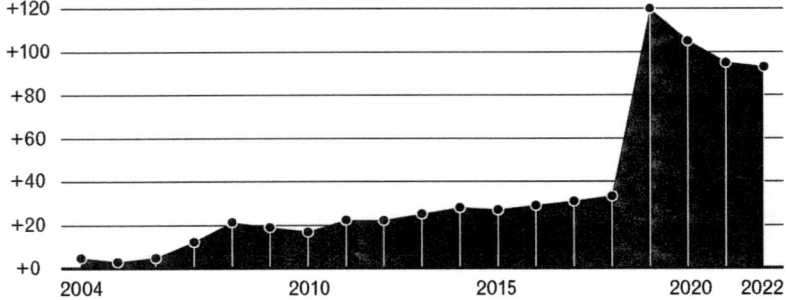

Adults' Time Spent at Home
U.S., Change in Minutes per Day Since 2003

Source: Patrick Sharkey, "Homebound: The Long-Term Rise in Time Spent at Home Among U.S. Adults," *Sociological Science* 11, no. 4 (January 2024): 553–78.

my own business. In my graduating class, there was only one other person who did that. Kids back then were less risk-aggressive, and a unicorn was still a fantastical being. Rather than become an entrepreneur, the smart money joined Intel, Deloitte, or a giant regional bank. I decided to buck the trend.

I was inspired by a class I took on brand strategy taught by David Aaker, generally considered the father of modern branding. I loved how brands were emotional and led to irrational purchases and above-market margins. *This is what I want to do with my life*, I thought. I told David I planned to start a business based on his class, and did he want to join me? Hell no, he said. So, with a friend who was good at the operations side, I launched Prophet, a brand strategy firm. I proceeded to pitch Yamaha Motor, which wanted to reinvigorate the Yamaha brand among younger Americans. Great, they said. What followed was a case study in slapstick improv. A friend created some credible graphics. Another friend worked at Bain, so I asked him, "How much would Bain charge?" He told me. I halved the number, though it was still exorbitant. "They'll never pay us that," my partner said. At the time I was living in a $220-a-month apartment in the Rockridge section of Oakland. Weeks later, I opened the mailbox to find a check from Yamaha Motors America representing one-third of the total due. I remember looking around, thinking, *Have I just committed fraud?* and *Am I about to get arrested?* It felt illegal, like I'd just fooled the world. But Yamaha stayed a client for years and we did a bunch of projects together. Two years after our founding, David Aaker joined Prophet as vice chairman. Thirty years later, he's still there, along with four hundred other people.

As you're starting out, if you're not in rooms where you don't belong, or doing things that make you feel you're out over your skis, the chances of your success exponentially decrease. Everything I'd done then I was unqualified for: attending UCLA, working at Morgan Stanley, and now starting my own strategy firm despite having zero experience in marketing or consulting. That didn't stop me from cold-calling companies and offering up my services. The world's most qualified, impressive people have one thing in common: they weren't qualified to do what they did. I've met my share of tech billionaires. They're impressive people, but less impressive than you think. Taking risks, being willing to feel like an imposter, is a key attribute of professional success—and masculinity.

Prophet was kind of successful right out of the gate. In 1997, we decided to incubate several e-commerce firms in the basement of Prophet's office, as that's what an MBA with a shaved head did in the nineties in San Francisco. I was raising money, starting e-commerce companies. I was beginning to hit my stride with the winds of processing power and the internet at my back, with luck and timing on my side.

FAIL FAST

"Never give up" tends to be the battle cry in America, especially in commencement addresses. Jesus, what bullshit. Entrepreneurs aren't voted into the hall of fame unless they have a story about mortgaging their house to make payroll or cleaning the first apartments rented on the platform. Sir James Dyson made 5,126 prototypes of his bagless vacuum cleaner, only to be rejected by every manufacturer in the UK. Jack Ma was rejected by Harvard ten times. Grit is great. Perseverance is a virtue. But, narratively, it's overrated. Greatness is a function not just of grit but of talent, luck, where and when you are born . . . and knowing when to quit.

Quitting is also a virtue. In fact, it's a necessity. The most successful prehistoric peoples were willing to leave a place when they observed a decline in prey or a change in the water. Most CEOs have one thing in common: they are quitters. Specifically, your career trajectory will be steeper if every several years you switch jobs. Strangers, from a distance, find you more attractive than coworkers, who can't help but look at you through the lens of when you joined the firm. The smart money quits fast.

In the mid-1990s, Prophet was on fire. We'd built the first websites for Williams Sonoma and Levi Strauss & Co. I was gaining a lot of intellectual capital around how to build winning e-commerce platforms. But I couldn't hold on to my best employees, who were getting picked off by start-ups and tech consulting firms. I decided to plug some of Prophet's revenues into a new business.

My idea: create the Williams Sonoma of pet supplies. (I had a dog, which clearly made me an expert in retail.) The pet retail channel back then was split between two kinds of retailers—big box stores (Walmart, Petco, PetSmart), and danker, smaller mom-and-pop stores that smelled bad; e.g., like parakeets. I went into business with an old business school classmate named Ian. I was creative; Ian could sell. I was all over the place; Ian was emotionless, organized, and even robotic. As someone who's always five minutes away from losing his apartment keys, I needed him. Ian and I named our new venture Aardvark, since the biggest online distribution channel back then listed its stores alphabetically, and Aardvark would bust out of the gate strong. Pretty soon we were doing $20,000 a month in e-commerce, making us, bizarrely, one of the one hundred most successful e-commerce sites in the world.

A publicly traded company, Utopia, offered to buy Ian and me out for $3 million in stock. For six months, I badgered Ian to close the deal, but he insisted on half of the $3 million in cash, the rest in stock. *But, Ian, this is e-commerce*, I kept saying. *You and I are going to the moon!* Finally I gave in, since Ian was smarter than me, and we got our $1.5 million in cash. Basically, I had tripled my money in eighteen months—one of the better investments I've made on an IRR basis (short for "internal rate of return," which measures the profitability of an investment), since within the year Utopia folded, our stock now worthless.

Around that time, I attended a seminar at Kleiner Perkins at which the VC and investor John Doerr said the internet was all about time-savings, especially for men. *How can I save time for men?*

I thought, realizing that *men are terrible at giving gifts*. Thanks to investments from Sequoia Capital, Chanel, and Presidio, I launched 911 Gifts with the homey tagline *The right gift right away*. Users went onto our website, typed in the name and demographics of the recipient, and were greeted with everything from a cashmere sleep mask to a chocolate body paint kit. They checked one, and we sent it off.

Months later, I was at a wedding in San Francisco. In those days, guests would sit around pretending to enjoy the spectacle of the newlyweds tearing open their gifts. One the bride unwrapped looked familiar. "Oh wow," she said, "this is beautiful." She flipped it over, scanned the label. "Huh," she called out to the (male) gift-giver, "so you thought of me at the very last minute?" She was joking, a.k.a., she was hurt and pissed.

Some moments are sadistically illuminating. There I was, running Prophet, advising some of the world's biggest companies on how to manage their brands, and I'd picked a company name that (a) evoked male haste and indifference, and (b) offended recipients. Good going, Scott. We immediately rebranded to RedEnvelope, referring to a custom across Asian cultures of handing over red envelopes stuffed with cash during social and family gatherings, holidays, and weddings. Red envelopes were believed to confer good luck.

The company CEO, also a board member, was a hugely successful VC. The two of us clashed immediately. I thought he was an asshat and know-nothing (the difference between being right and being effective hadn't yet clicked for me). I wasn't shy about letting him know this, either. I was headed to the airport after a vituperative board meeting when he and one of his lieutenants called me. I'd been kicked off the board.

The ensuing controversy attracted a lot of press. *The New York Times* even described me as "spunky." Naturally, I handled the whole thing as poorly as possible. An angry young man with too much time on his hands and some money is dangerous. I embarked on a full-scale proxy fight, the goal being to replace the CEO and all the board members. I didn't get the votes. Basically, despite spending half a million dollars of my own money, I was ejected from the band I'd started, while the markets were signaling I was batshit crazy and should go away. It was a professional low point.

I literally had no idea what to do next. I decided to get angry again.

After raising an additional $10 million to $20 million, I was now RedEnvelope's largest shareholder. I retook control of the company and the board and put in a new CEO. My return evoked the time General MacArthur returned to the Philippines in 1944, though in my case I and everyone in my environs proceeded to get shot repeatedly in the face. Negative momentum is a real thing.

First, the new CEO overestimated margins by a thousand basis points, causing RedEnvelope's stock to drop from 14 to 7 in one day, incensing investors. This was followed by a longshoreman's strike, which left much of our holiday merchandise imprisoned on a cargo ship off the coast of Long Beach. With the credit crisis taking hold, Wells Fargo took the opportunity to slash our credit line. Then a software glitch in RedEnvelope's fulfillment center meant twelve thousand gifts got shipped to the wrong addresses. Stuff like this can kill you. Within ninety days we'd gone from a stock trading at $7 to Chapter 11. Ultimately, I lost everything: a bunch of my own money, but also ten years of emotional and psychological involvement and jobs for two hundred or so employees. To this day, whenever someone says the words "red" or "envelope," the small of my back starts sweating and I want to throw up.

RedEnvelope was my "learning business," my biggest, most public professional disaster. I didn't know that, while winning is the best thing, the second-best thing is quitting/failing fast. For example, in 1999, I founded an e-commerce incubator, Brand Farm. Nine months later, I shut it down. Didn't matter. Why? Again, nine months. Fail fast = twenty-four months or less. The alternative—failing excruciatingly slowly over a ten-year period—is the absolute pits.

NOTHING VENTURED

Anything that offers substantial rewards comes with risk, a high likelihood of failure. Which means you'll need to make several appearances at the plate before you connect with the ball. The top scorers in the Premier League miss half their shots. Great players, like great entrepreneurs and leaders, see the ball go wide, shake their heads, and move on. If you want to be successful, you will likely need to quit the majority of your jobs, homes, and investments. Your jobs, locale, investment, and relationships are commitments, not suicide pacts.

What gets labeled "overnight successes" rarely are, and the best way to become an overnight success is to work your ass off for thirty years. Most hugely successful entrepreneurs don't hit it on their first venture.

WHEN TO WALK AWAY

The challenge is knowing which part of the script you're in. Are you at the moment where, if you dig in, your perseverance will pay off? Or are you somewhere in the first hundred minutes of the movie, experiencing just one of a string of failures? Math offers a hint: You're likely to experience many more failures than successes, so if you know nothing else about your situation, be open to the notion (*gasp*) that this may be one of the failures. And, most important, that you and humanity will survive it.

Quitting often requires walking away from years of invested time and capital. Our brains aren't wired for this—we're unable to recognize that sunk costs are . . . sunk. One study asked participants to imagine they had bought nonrefundable tickets for two different weekend trips, one costing $100, the other $50, but they'd inadvertently bought them for the same date. The $50 trip would be more fun, they were told. Which trip would they take? Irrationally, 54 percent of people said they would go on the $100 trip. We hate walking away from an investment.

Semi-quitting (i.e., diversifying) is a critical skill in good times as well. On the boards of start-ups, at every subsequent round of financing, I encourage management and employees to take some money off the table. And, increasingly, this is an option for small-growth firms. It's amazing how the power pendulum has swung from VCs to founders. When I was starting companies in the nineties, VCs and bankers wouldn't tolerate this. "That would send the wrong signal—aren't you in this to win?" Pro tip: if you have 80+ percent of your net worth in one asset and people try to stop you from diversifying, they do not have your best interests at heart.

HIGH COUNSEL

I'm not suggesting you be reckless, get divorced, and head for Key West. Even Cersei Lannister had a high counsel and a hand (senior adviser). Spoiler alert: she stopped listening to them. Everyone needs their own high counsel, and you should not make any big decision without the benefit of their input. It's difficult to read the label from inside the bottle. However, the thing that often holds back people who are emotionally strong and talented is their hesitancy to leave, to quit. It's a vastly underrated strength. When Liverpool FC manager Jürgen Klopp announced he was leaving when his team was in first place because he didn't feel he had the energy he owed the team, the fans loved him for his integrity and his stature was enhanced. That's a form of strength.

SHAME

Nobody is paying as much attention to your failures as you are, so fear them but don't let them paralyze you. When you do fail, don't feel you need to excuse your failures or blame others. Being gracious in victory is admirable. What's harder, but can pay greater dividends, is being gracious in failure. Express gratitude to everyone who believed in you, and demonstrate grace to those who didn't.

Shame and fear of embarrassment often hold people back from leaving . . . and leading a better life. Carl Sagan's insight helps liberate me from that angst: "We are mites on a plum on a planet circling an unremarkable star on the outskirts of an ordinary galaxy which contains 400 billion other stars and is one of 100 billion other galaxies." Nobody you care about or who cares about you will be alive in a hundred years. Nobody will remember your successes or failures. To let fear devour your short time here is to not understand the most basic law of the universe: your insignificance. Why would any of us not enjoy ourselves and not love others with abandon?

> **Note:** *Don't be afraid to quit. Failing fast is better than failing over a long period.*

AMERICAN MADE

I constantly humblebrag that I was raised by a single immigrant mother who lived and died as a secretary. But the truth is I was born on third base. My parents got me to first base before I was born by immigrating to the United States. This took courage, desire, and a dose of selfishness. Both left families that needed them. My mom left London when her two youngest siblings were still in an orphanage.

A lot of success isn't your fault. My patriotism is a function of the fact that I'm a white, heterosexual male who was born and came of age in the right place and the right time, had access to the elite California education system for not much money, and, despite mediocre grades, got a job at Morgan Stanley, which gave me the credibility to get admitted to Berkeley, which, as the internet (a uniquely American thing) was dawning, gave me the credibility to live in San Francisco and raise $100 million in the next six to eight years for my start-ups, providing so much opportunity and growth that the only real talent I needed was proficiency at surfing a one-hundred-foot wave. Not only could that never happen outside the United States, it probably couldn't have happened in another city, and it may never have happened if I hadn't been a young white guy.

Yes, there's surfing elsewhere. But there's a difference between riding a monster wave and a wave in a mostly motionless lake. The two other regions where the greatest economic opportunities exist are Europe and China. The former is overregulated, hasn't seen much growth, and risks turning into an open-air museum. China today is experiencing high youth unemployment, workplace disillusionment, and a mismatch between high-end jobs and applicants; as of 2023, more than half of all Chinese citizens ages twenty-five to twenty-nine are unmarried.

Part of maturing and becoming a man is acknowledging your blessings. I overcame some early obstacles and today I'm a self-made man. I'm also American made: born on third base, later crammed into 28 percent of the population (white males with graduate degrees), adjacent to most of the capital inside the world's most prosperous nation. My reductive analysis: I'd rather be average in America than good in Europe. Also, the United States is the best place to make money; Europe is the best place to spend it.

This made me realize (a) it's wonderful to be American, and (b) some percentage of my success is random, lucky, and based on happenstance. This dawned on me in my forties, along with the recognition that I needed to start creating those same opportunities for others, to make sure the drawbridge hadn't closed.

> **Note:** *Part of maturing and becoming a man means acknowledging your blessings—and creating opportunities for others.*

The anger and frustration many younger Americans feel today is legitimate. They're up against economic realities that their parents and grandparents simply were not: rising inflation, soaring housing prices, unbridled student debt, AI labor disruptions, and a climate crisis that could someday make all of it moot. The culture is marked by loutishness and division. The world's most profitable companies are guided by algorithms that churn up incendiary content and feed off of us enraging and shit-posting one another and our government.

Speedballed by those algorithms, young people today are the first generation in American history to not do better than their parents. They lack the same opportunities to meet potential mates. A lot of factors are at play, including less purchasing power with increased costs, political division, greater health consciousness, declining church attendance, phone addiction, and an absence of so-called third spaces (public spaces that are neither work nor home)—a perfect storm of young people *not* connecting and mating. In England, more than four hundred nightclubs have closed in the past five years, representing more than a third of the total. Where, then, are young people supposed to meet? Along with student debt, young people worry about getting sick, the cost of healthcare in general, and finding a good doctor who hasn't gone boutique (good luck). Housing in major cities, and even renting, is an unattainable stretch. As smart, talented, and hardworking as their parents were at their age, young people can't get into the same-quality colleges, higher education having figured out a way to extract more money by artificially constraining supply, thereby forcing these kids to attend lesser places that are—wait for it—exponentially more expensive.

Moreover, attacks come in daily, from all sides—economic, psychological, legislative. Young people face a food industrial complex determined to make them obese and diabetic, the better to hand them over to the pharmaceutical industrial complex and a world of statins that increase longevity, giving rise to additional panic about the financial and emotional costs of living ten to twenty years longer than their grandparents. Meanwhile, they're reminded three hundred times a day that (a) they and their neighbors hate each other politically, and (b) everyone but them seems to be on a Gulfstream or at a VIP party in St. Barts. According to a 2025 Harvard Youth Poll involving two thousand respondents, four out of ten Americans under thirty report that they're "barely getting by" economically; only 16 percent say they're doing "well," much less "very well." Fewer than half feel a sense of community, and only 15 percent believe the United States is heading in the right direction, with only 19 percent trusting the federal government to reliably do the right thing. That's the whole shooting match right there, a five-alarm fire for the United States. If young people don't feel good about their country, they'll storm the castle, and the country won't survive. Their arguments are legitimate—my generation has not paid it forward.

Some would argue there's more opportunity elsewhere. But the United States still offers the best economic circumstances and the highest rates of income mobility (the ability to migrate from the lowest to the uppermost quintile), also the most agency, though there's less here than there used to be. What's changed is perspective, the

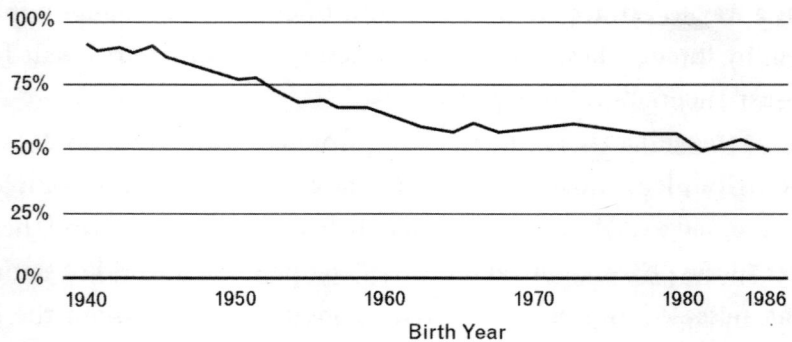

Share of 30-Year-Olds Earning More Than Their Parents Did at Age 30
U.S., by Birth Year

Source: Raj Chetty et al., "The Fading American Dream: Trends in Absolute Income Mobility Since 1940," *Science* 356, no. 6336 (April 2017): 398–406, Fig. 1.

way the wealth benchmark has become more pronounced and finely diced, how daily it gets shoved in your face how incredibly well others are doing compared with you. (Note: you're not even seeing the top 1 percent online because they, wary of coming across as obnoxious and clueless, don't post on social media. Anyone posting a close-up of their jet likely doesn't own one.) Younger people are still lucky to live here. The smartest thing I ever did was being born in the United States. Even as the son of a single immigrant mother, I got access to a free, world-class education as a kid and later came of age in an era when the United States was building more shareholder value within a seven-mile radius of San Francisco than existed in all of Europe, not to mention how our tax code favors small businesses. America celebrates risk and risk-takers, and tolerates failure. Seriously, where else on the planet can someone like me start nine companies and not be flogged publicly for the failures?

Today, the least patriotic people are those who are most blessed and who lead extraordinary and rewarding lives, specifically tech bros. My advice: Go on a short California road trip, starting in San Diego and ending in San Francisco. Out the window there's Qualcomm, and in L.A. there's SpaceX, Snap, and Netflix. Farther north is Meta, Alphabet, and Salesforce. Together, these companies are worth trillions of dollars. Then something happens. Once you reach Canada, everything stops, just as it does on the southern tip when you hit Mexico and find a radically different culture, society, and set of laws. Would today's tech bros be billionaires in Calgary or San Miguel de Allende? Strongly doubt it, yet the bros are among the first to shit-post the United States and bang on about how fucked-up it is.

I'm not sure young Americans altogether appreciate their blessings and opportunities relative to living elsewhere, or how many people have made sacrifices to ensure those rights and protections. Send a hundred college sophomores to the worst, most embattled parts of the world. Interview them afterward. See what they say. Most if not all will be on the first flight home.

WHAT IT'S ALL FOR

When my mom's cancer came back a third time, I was thirty-eight and professionally more successful. I helped her sell her condo in Westwood and moved her into a two-bedroom apartment on a golf course in Summerlin, a Las Vegas suburb. Among my first clients at Prophet was Williams Sonoma. I asked them for a discount, and they gave me 40 percent off. Taking advantage, I furnished her new place in one of its brands, Pottery Barn—at the time it might as well have been Hermès. I was finally making enough money to do things like that for her. It was an incredibly rewarding feeling, a big moment to be able to do that for my mom, who had always worked so hard to support me. She could retire now and not freak out more than she was already about being sick and not working. It was one of the first times I remember feeling like a real man.

At thirty-eight, I had flexibility and money. I was teaching only a couple of classes at NYU, could take time off, and was able to do my "activist investor" stuff remotely. So I moved in with my mom, serving as her comfort. It made sense: I was her only family. Almost immediately we received a note from her apartment complex, Del Webb Active Adult Community. It had come to their attention that my mom was cohabitating with a man under the age of fifty, which violated . . . whatever. I walked over to the office. "I'm not cohabitating," I said. "My mom is dying. I'm her son. I'm here to take care of her." They backed down. A note of humor in the overall grimness.

Two things topped my mom's bucket list: saying goodbye to her family in London and dying at home. The first was easy. She was sick but not prohibitively, and I got her to the UK and back, thanks to my half sister, Asheley, who was working at the time for an airline and finagled an upgrade. The second, arranging for her to die at home, was harder. Death is persnickety, shitty at keeping appointments. I didn't know if my mom would last one month or six months, though it was within that time frame. The doctors made a plan for super-aggressive chemo. The five-year survival rate was around 6 percent—basically it was a science experiment that might ultimately add thirty-five days to her life. My mom was pragmatic. Instead of fighting back, she chose comfort.

It's brutal watching someone you love being eaten alive by stomach cancer. The harshness of it was eye-opening. I couldn't imagine anyone willing to go through what she was going through. My mom's illness made eating difficult, and she suffered with constant nausea and pain. She endured it all without complaining. During the day, the two of us hung out together. I oversaw her nutrition and morphine. We both loved TV and watched a lot of shows—*Frasier, Jeopardy!, Everybody Loves Raymond, Friends*. We looked at photos and exchanged stories. I didn't want to leave anything unsaid. It was impossible to say "I love you" too much or tell her how much I admired her. I would sit next to her on the couch, hold her hand, weep, and tell her how sad I was that this was happening and that she had to go through it.

At the end of their lives, I believe parents want two things: the knowledge their family loves them immensely, and that their love and parenting gave their kids the skills and confidence to add value to the world and live rewarding lives.

Her friends were great. They would visit for a few days, sometimes weeks at a time, and help with bathing and changing my mom. My mom's old boss, a very successful executive twenty years younger than her with his own family, would board a plane at LAX, fly to Las Vegas every two months, and sit beside her for an hour. By that point, my mom was retching into a plastic bag every twenty minutes. It would have been easy for him not to do that, to make excuses, but he didn't. He was goodness, decency in action.

My mom would fall asleep at seven or eight p.m. I'd drive to the

Strip and get drunk with entrepreneurs who were starting cigar bars and restaurants. Then I drove home to Summerlin and fell asleep. Knowing I needed to have my own life and space, I ring-fenced my time. Every Thursday, I flew to NYC or Miami for the weekend to maintain my friendships and keep my professional life alive, aware whatever I'd achieved was a testament to the positive environment in which my mom raised me. During one trip to Miami, I met my now wife. If I hadn't left, today I wouldn't be married or have two sons, and neither would my mom likely have had grandkids.

Given three months, my mom lived another four. Unfortunately, one Sunday I flew back, and she had passed two hours earlier. I wish I'd been there but would not change it. Had I not had some semblance of a life I would have been less pleasant to be around and maybe less available to my mom emotionally.

When you die, it doesn't matter how nice your home is. If at your exit you're surrounded only by strangers under bright lights, it's a disappointment. Of course, this isn't an option for many people, but the goal is to die at home, surrounded by people who love you. You need to live well to die well, with a life filled with meaningful relationships where you were generous with people. My mom had an eighth-grade education, was divorced, and worked her whole life as a secretary. She drew her last breath at home, comfortable and surrounded by people who loved her immensely.

Today, she'd be pleased to know I have a son who looks like her and whose middle name is, like hers, Sylvia.

She, along with my wife and boys, are why I've worked so hard.

chapter 5

HEALTH

In the early 1950s, two mountaineers and fitness freaks came up with the Kraus-Weber tests—a set of exercises targeting flexibility and arm and core strength. These were administered to seven thousand kids globally, including four thousand from the United States. Nearly 60 percent of American kids failed, versus 8 percent of Europeans. The findings depressed President Eisenhower enough so that he soon rolled out the Presidential Fitness Test for middle and high school students—pull-ups, sit-ups, standing broad jump, shuttle run, 50-yard dash, softball throw, and 600-yard run. The goal was to encourage physical activity nationwide and make kids feel better about themselves. More than a half century later, the program disbanded.

The PFT wasn't perfect, but it was a shot in the right direction. When did we decide aspirational fitness—and getting stronger and more disciplined about everything you do in life—was no different from fat-shaming? When did we decide obesity was more about finding your truth instead of finding type-2 diabetes and cardiovascular disease? The progressive left ignored Covid-19 data showing obesity was correlated with both increased severity and morbidity of symptoms while contributing to 30 percent of all hospitalizations.

I get it: some people are born big. Obesity is heritable in individuals at rates ranging from 25 to 80 percent. Other individuals living in food deserts are forced to rely on fast food as their easiest and most affordable food source. Hormonal, medical, cultural, and psychological factors play a part. Born with different genetics, I could have easily ended up overweight—all that shepherd's pie. Eating healthily is expensive and so is cooking from scratch every night at home. Jack in the Box is the most economically efficient way for a single mom to funnel calories into her son. Obese people shouldn't be shamed or bullied, but neither should empathy become enablement.

In the United States, obesity has been normalized. A medical condition responsible for $173 billion in American medical costs is big business. Plus-size clothing is a $330 billion industry, expected to rise to more than $400 billion by 2030, with others profiting mightily, too, such as multinational food companies, digital health companies hawking nutrition and fitness tracking, diabetes and GLP-1 medications, knee and hip replacements, kidney dialysis, and statins. Contrast this to Japan, which has the lowest percentage of obese and overweight adults—4.5 percent—of all rich countries globally, compared with 42 percent of Americans. Japanese kids learn early on to stop eating when they're 80 percent full. By law, every Japanese elementary school keeps a nutritionist on staff. Strict rules govern that lunches and snacks are homemade and meet nutritional guidelines. "Broccoli," a Japanese first-grader might say when asked about a food they like—compared with the sugary, ultraprocessed lunches served across U.S. schools.

Our national unfitness has security ramifications. American armed service enrollment numbers are down dramatically. This is attributable to a number of factors, including poor test scores, widespread distrust of institutions and government on the part of potential applicants, and better economic opportunities elsewhere. Ninety percent of all applicants to the Army, Navy, Marines, Air Force, and Coast Guard are between the ages of eighteen and twenty-four. For many, though, the fitness test is disqualifying—one in three applicants is too out of shape. Around 77 percent require a waiver, the primary reason being weight/poor fitness, mental health issues, and drug abuse. If you're in decent shape, you can leave an army recruitment office with a four-year assignment. The service pays for college. You'll get a job immediately at a good salary. What would it mean for the U.S. military, healthcare costs, depression/anxiety rates, and increased mating opportunities if a significant percentage of the U.S. population became healthier in their diet, weight, and lifestyle?

Physicality should begin early. Boys are like dogs—they need to run and get exhausted, roughhouse, wrestle, build and smash things, sweat, whale against other bodies and objects. On the other end, dads should kiss their sons, hold their hands, hug them good night—model what fully functioning men have it within us to do and be, the affection and care humans share with those they love. The bad news is that from 2013 to 2023, the participation in sports of boys ages six to seventeen dropped by almost ten points, from around 50 to 41 percent. Among Black boys, the figure dropped to 35 percent.

Physicality implies a willingness to engage in the physical world. The inability to endure rejection in the physical world pushes boys and young men to lower-risk barriers of entry online. A bad habit.

Every boy and young man grows up wanting to express his masculinity. Most do this through rebellions large and small. If rebellion is your thing, don't attack your parents. Rise up instead against the corporate platforms that are making obscene amounts of money from making you addicted to their products. The axis of evil isn't Iran, Iraq, and North Korea—it's the American industrial food, medical, and pharmaceutical complexes. The deepest-pocketed, most talented companies in the world profit mightily by making you indignant, overweight, unhealthy, addicted, and at war with America and your fellow citizens. These companies are and should be your enemies. Decide instead to be a fit, patriotic, patient, disciplined, loving man—then work toward becoming that person.

Richard Reeves once quoted the headmaster of a private UK boys' school who said his mission was to cultivate men who would be "acceptable at a dance and invaluable in a shipwreck." The citation is a century old. It's still true. Start now.

STRONG

We are happiest when in motion and surrounded by others. A decent proxy for your success will be your ratio of sweating to watching others sweat. It's not about being skinny or ripped but committing to being strong physically and mentally. Walking into any conference room or bar and believing that, if shit got real, you could defend yourself there gives you confidence (note: *don't* do this).

The most common trait among CEOs isn't the colleges they went to, or their ethnicity, or the ability to get by on two hours of sleep; it's that many exercise four to five times a week. If you adopt a single CEO trait, I would strongly advise taking this one to heart. If you were offered a drug that was guaranteed to make you less depressed, give you focus and make you think more clearly, make you eat better and drink more water, and increase your dating pool, wouldn't you take that drug?

> **Note:** *Walking into any conference room or bar and believing that, if shit got real, he could defend himself gives a young man confidence.* (**Extra note:** Don't do this.)

ANTIDEPRESSANT

Of the three legs of the keep-Scott-sane stool—nutrition, sleep, exercise—I excel most at exercise. For the past forty years, I've worked out four times a week. I credit my dad for hauling me into the garage when I was eleven and showing me his Royal Navy manual: burpees, pull-ups, push-ups, bicep curls, dead lifts. I got into it immediately, as it drew us closer. So did the long runs we took on the beach whenever I visited him and Linda; he had no idea what else to do with me.

I've passed this habit on to my own boys. Alec, my eldest, is away at boarding school, and every night at nine or ten, he and I do a ten-minute Royal Navy workout on Zoom. It brings us closer, as it did my dad and me.

Exercise and time with my family are my two antidepressants. Not trying to be Hallmark Channel here, but I get seriously down or scream at my kids if I don't sweat three to five times a week.

I work out at Equinox, which is $250 a month and is no different than New York Sports Club ($50 a month), except the guys are hotter, and women wear seriously fabulous athleisure. This makes Equinox, for me, an incredible value, as I feel hotter and more fashionable, via association, two to three times a week. I wear headphones, as I don't want to talk to anybody. The last sentence is a delusion—I believe it but know deep down it's just not true. People want to speak to me at school, work (sometimes), at conferences (rarely), but nobody wants to talk to me at Equinox. When I went to sign up for a membership, the sales associate wouldn't even look me in the eye, just swiped my Amex and told me to download the app.

A lot of new research shows how exercise helps your muscles and enzymes recover. According to the Mayo Clinic, regular exercise has a staggering number of other benefits, too, including weight control, increased energy, an elevation of HDL, or "good" cholesterol, better sleep, and a better sex life. I look better. I feel better. I like myself more. I feel better walking up the stairs. I feel stronger, more successful, more focused, more in charge.

Until recently, I did CrossFit. Now I have a personal trainer. I get it: most people who work all day and come home to cook dinner and take care of kids don't have that luxury. Absent personal training, there are a ton of great fitness apps out there. As you get older, it's more about injury prevention. To be clear, relationships (including with yourself) matter more than anything. But a close second is your relationship with the only temple you'll ever have: your body.

The goal is to start early, to develop and refine the exercise muscle when you're young; it's easier to slow the decline that way. Trying to get into shape at sixty after a lifetime of being in bad shape is almost impossible. After fifty, it's hard putting on muscle. Choose an exercise you enjoy or don't hate; otherwise you won't show up. As for other stuff, I'm not someone who gets up at four a.m., does a cold plunge, listens to exactly thirty-three seconds of Bach's Minuet in G Minor, gets into a sauna, and meditates for an hour. Though I know I would benefit from mindfulness, I just don't do it. Spending solo time with my dogs and computer and listening and learning after my family has gone to bed gives me some peace.

> **Note:** *Be and stay fit—it has cascading effects on all other areas of your life.*

MIND THE GAP

The biggest secret to working out is not thinking about doing it but *doing* it.

When I began resistance training, it filled a hole of insecurity in me that I wasn't muscular enough. It was also good for my mental health. CrossFit classes offer accountability, community, and support. I stopped going last year and today have a personal trainer. It's not like he knows anything I don't. What he can do, uniquely, is arrange for us to meet in my garage on Sunday mornings. This cuts through my procrastination, my habit of putting exercising off until I quite literally can't do it; e.g., I have a Zoom, or it's dinner, or I have to get to the airport.

It's a universal truth that everyone enjoys having worked out, past tense, the problem being that the hours leading up to it are horrific.

If someone handed me a pill that guaranteed I would never have to work out again but could still realize the benefits of working out, I would pocket the bottle. The gap between evaluating when I should work out versus doing it is what kills momentum. Collapsing the moment separating "should" and "do" has been a revelation.

Another is recognizing that spending twenty to thirty minutes doing half a dozen weight-bearing exercises with intense music blaring in my ears is as good as, if not better than, going to Equinox, checking in, changing, figuring out that day's workout, doing it, stretching, showering, and going home. So I created a dwarf facsimile of a gym in my home studio with dumbbells, a kettlebell, and a bench press. If I go hard, I can do a decent workout in a half hour or less, three to four times a week. It's all about intensity and frequency.

> **Note:** *Nothing kills momentum faster than knowing you "should" exercise . . . and putting it off. Mind the gap—do it.*

BULKING UP

I didn't discover sports and weightlifting until college. I made the lightweight crew team despite being only a mediocre athlete. Told I was strong enough to make the heavyweight team, I was given access to the UCLA training staff.

A nutritionist changed my diet completely. When you're nineteen, all you need is protein. Cholesterol and salt don't really matter for most young people—they can easily turn a McDonald's Spicy McCrispy and a large fries into muscle. Creatine wasn't around, but milk, bananas, peanut butter sandwiches, and Top Ramen (my luxury) were. They were cost-effective, too—I spent 60 cents a day on food. Then, on Sundays, the entire crew team would descend on Sizzler, where for $3.99 we gorged on steak, Malibu chicken (whatever that is), and the all-you-can-eat salad bar. We'd show up at four p.m.

for meal #1, leave, hang out in Westwood, maybe see a movie, and circle back to Sizzler for meal #2 at eight o'clock. That's roughly eight thousand calories for four bucks. Eating there twice was bold, but no manager was about to eject two dozen very tall, two-hundred-pound UCLA students, many of whom were broke. Eighteen months later, I'd gone from skinny to built. My new physique, and the medication I was taking for my skin, made me *a UCLA athlete*. Women noticed.

Until then, I'd relied on humor to attract women. Suddenly it was about the way I looked. For this reason, I've always thought of strength and muscles and fitness positively. A ridiculous amount of my self-confidence grew from all three.

When I moved to NYC, I was bored and depressed. I found stretching and hitting helped, and I began practicing boxing and yoga, the former at a downtown boxing club popular with models, investment bankers, and depressed professors. I would beat the shit out of that speed bag. My boxing trainer, a twentysomething kid named Anthony, convinced me I had a "gift" as a pugilist, probably because I was paying him $80 an hour. I knew he was lying, but that didn't stop me from believing him. We decided I should participate in their quarterly boxing tournament.

A. Great. Idea.

I had been training like a maniac and felt good, confident even. So, twenty years ago, Scott "Prof G" Galloway entered the ring. I was six-foot-two, 188, and my opponent was five-foot-eight, 191. Facing each other, in the center of the ring, it looked as if Ichabod Crane was about to get it on with Mike Tyson's big brother. *No problem, I've got this ... Anthony said I have a gift.* My freakishly long arms would keep the elder Iron Mike at bay. The bell rang, and my first thought was how bright it was.

The brightness was a function of my being flat on my back just after the bell rang, approximately seventeen seconds that I don't remember and will never get back, and the temporary loss of function in the orbicularis oculi muscle and my facial nerve—the pathway that controls blinking. I thought I saw Nana—what I'd have called my dead grandmother had I ever met her. Despite headgear that could deflect a laser, I'd been hit hard, and after returning from temporary unconsciousness, I couldn't feel the left side of my face. It appears speed bags that hit back render me an awful boxer. Men are just wired to misinterpret signals that inflate our confidence, so we'll hunt bigger prey and approach potential mates. Sixteen years later, my nose still veers to the right. In sum, the most common mistake in strategy is believing your competitor is a speed bag and doesn't observe, calculate, and hit back.

Yoga? It was mostly an excuse to meet women. The studio was called Muti. Eighty percent of the students were hot, easy-to-approach women. I ended up dating two yoga instructors. For a man who doesn't know many people in New York and wants to clear his head and get some exercise (and go on dates), I highly recommend yoga.

For me, fitness is more a need than a want. I've noticed my mild anger and depression issues are directly correlated to whether I've worked out that day or week. Not an anomaly here: along with boosting mood, lowering appetite, improving sleep, and lowering the risks of stroke, heart disease, dementia, and a bunch of cancers, studies show exercise also lowers levels of adrenaline and cortisol (a.k.a. your stress hormones), while ramping up endorphins (a.k.a. your body's natural painkillers). Exercise can even help with addiction by decreasing drug-seeking behaviors in people of all ages. Any exercise works. For people struggling to find the right meds to treat their depression, a 2024 study shows that exercise is the best nonpharmacological treatment out there. Also? Women appreciate fitness in men. It signals a man can show up, is disciplined and committed, and cares about the way he looks, which are the same attributes that make a man successful professionally and personally as a partner and father. I can't see how any man can't find a way to introduce some form of fitness in his life—stretching, running, biking, walking more. Stronger, you become kinder. You feel better about yourself. You're more attractive to potential mates.

The downside is that I still struggle with body dysmorphia. There's a photo of me from fifteen years ago. I was six-two, two hundred pounds, taking a shit-ton of creatine, and looking like Lou Ferrigno's tensely smiling younger brother. Did I need to be that big? If so, why wasn't I wearing it better? What was the point? I remember thinking I looked scrawny and needed to put on ten more pounds of muscle. In sum, six decades in, much like a lot of other people, I still don't feel totally comfortable in my body, but I accept it.

> **Note:** *Fitness sends a signal that you can show up, are disciplined and committed, and take pride in who you are; i.e., the same attributes that make a man successful professionally and personally as a partner and father.*

GETTING TO IT

Getting your body moving is essential for immediate and long-term health. In my experience, the best exercise translates to real-world situations—walking, hiking, raking leaves, sprinting to catch a flight. For the latest research, I asked fellow podcaster Andrew Huberman. His advice:

Lighting Up

Try to soak in sunlight first thing in the a.m. A recent study looked at light exposure during the day and at night among eighty thousand people. Those who took in fifteen to twenty minutes of bright light first thing after waking up had significantly improved mental health compared with those who didn't. Light even reduces the symptoms of people dealing with anxiety, depression, PTSD, and bipolar disorders. Not screen light or bedside lamp light, either—too weak. Sunlight is best, followed by a 10,000-lux lamp or ring light. Light during the night, though, can exacerbate preexisting mental health disorders.

Keep your bedroom dark, or buy a sleep mask. If you have trouble falling and staying asleep, odds are your evening light exposure has something to do with it. It's a simple, zero-cost adjustment.

Cardio

Moving your body is essential for immediate and long-term health. The literature tells us we should be walking more than we are. Broken down further: try to do three sessions of cardio a week, any format—running, biking, swimming. Just don't injure yourself. One workout should be longer, forty-five to sixty minutes, and involve a longer distance, where you're barely able to have a conversation. A second should be quicker, about a half hour where you push harder. A third should be brief, sprinting for ten to fifteen seconds anywhere from five to eight times, rest, and repeat. These shorter, faster bursts give you your VO_2 max (the maximum amount of oxygen you use during strenuous exercise) and help with conditioning and life (yard work, busting your ass to make a flight, helping your wife with her suitcase).

Weights

Resistance training is vital, too—it's less about aesthetics than it is about keeping your muscles healthy, and helping you improve your metabolism and maintain cognitive function (e.g., atrophy of the calves is linked to dementia). Go for a whole-body workout two to three times a week, three sets for every major muscle group—quads, triceps, biceps, etc.—an hour total. Or split things up: one day your legs, the next time your torso, the third time biceps, triceps, and shoulders. It's exciting putting on muscle, so resist the temptation to overdo it: go slow, don't get hurt, make sure you get the right rest and nutrition. Eighty to 90 percent of workouts should be 80 to 90 percent of what you can do. Don't go all out. Keep gas in the tank. Not every run has to end with a sprint.

Three days a week of cardio, a few hours of resistance training—that's it.

A big part of masculinity is about being the best, strongest version of yourself, someone who can help others. Strap on your oxygen mask first—you're useless as a protector if you're dead. This means taking care of yourself by getting annual physicals, and calling your doctor if something feels off, versus waiting to get nagged by your partner. I once had a meeting with one of the best, most perceptive investment bankers in history. He was always the smartest, most tactical guy in the room. Rumpled and cerebral, and lacking social skills, he was also overweight. Terrible blood pressure. He didn't take care of himself. Dead at sixty-one. Don't be him.

> **Note:** *You can't take care of others if you don't take care of yourself first. Get annual checkups, stay healthy.*

Teeth count, too. Coming out of the closet here: I have terrible dental hygiene; i.e., I brush my teeth once, usually twice, a day, and in six decades have flossed maybe a dozen times. In this era that's like saying you're a sex trafficker. I get my teeth cleaned every three months. After years of feeling shamed and infantilized by dentists and making windy promises that I'll change my ways, buy an electric toothbrush, floss three times a day for the rest of my life, I tell the hygienist to spare me the lecture. She laughs. At least I'm being honest, she says. My advice: Don't be like me. Floss.

INTO THE WOODS

Stepping outside is another fitness value-add. Being outside offers a bunch of positive benefits: it lowers blood pressure and heart rate, enhances immune function, and decreases the likelihood of diabetes and cardiovascular mortality. Exposure to sunlight increases testosterone levels in men, while trips to the park improve health outcomes and create resilience in children who've experienced trauma, abuse, and poverty. Spending two hours a week outside has been shown to significantly increase health and happiness. Some doctors prescribe spending time in nature. The Swedes have a word for this, *frilufsliv*, "living close to nature," and they offer tax breaks for companies with policies that encourage it. The biggest threat to this lifestyle? The crowding out of the outside world by our devices, consumed mostly in the inside world.

Meeting strangers and experiencing novel environments is fundamental to human growth. Our podcast producer once told me she was cultivating a practice of "say yes to everything." I loved this. The comfortable and the familiar are the harbingers of weakness and fear. Without rejection and awkwardness, you won't experience victory or true satisfaction . . . the feeling that you've achieved something.

A common saying in my youth: "Nothing good happens after two a.m." This was mostly true, as the "after" part usually involved (more) alcohol and chasing a high and an environment that peaked at midnight. The chase, if repeated too often, can begin to impair your ability to register progress during the day, which is key to your success at night. Simply put, it's all about what you do during the day. I believe this should be modified to "it's all about what you do outside of the home." The point of differentiation between those making a living and those having a significant impact will, I believe, be a function of their success in the physical presence of others.

> **Note:** *Get outside. Just fifteen minutes of sunlight in the morning helps your mental health.*

THE SCOTT METHOD

When friends ask if I'll mentor their sons, I always say yes. We focus on four things: fitness, nutrition, money, work. Master these and they'll be in a place to start exploring relationships.

It's worth repeating: many men think they have to be a mix of

Aristotle, Gandalf, and Mr. Miyagi from *The Karate Kid* to mentor a younger person. That's horseshit. The questions I get asked are easy, and a cat could give the advice I do.

I ask questions as mundane as: *When's the last time you ate a real meal? What do you eat and drink during an average day? Red Bull, Cheetos, sativa gummies? How do you think those might affect your body and brain? So . . . you work in retail, and/or you earn four hundred bucks a week at Chipotle? How much of that goes to online sports betting? A hundred dollars a week? That means you're spending a quarter of your income on gambling. How are your relationships? Are you dating? What's your relationship with your parents like? What about your relationship with yourself? What's your story? Do you have a plan, a blueprint, a map? If not, let's come up with one. You can adjust it, swap it out in six months or a year; nonetheless, you need one. Do you want to apply to junior college? Skip college, enter the workforce? Move out of your childhood bedroom and start having sex with strange women? First you need to make some money.*

Young men have a single source of capital: time. Where to find it? On their phones. By tracking their activities, we reallocate those hours to more productive places.

I'm eternally amazed by the number of college-age kids who live at home and who are convinced their parents are the enemy. Yes, your parents can be tone-deaf, uncool, a source of frustration, but give me a fucking break—they're not trying to undermine you or wreck your life. Unless home is a hellscape, and they're abusing you, assume everything they do comes from a good place. Don't want to obey house rules? Then stop taking your parents' money and find a fifth-floor walk-up. Accepting their support means taking their advice.

Next, we unlock their phones. Not so I can judge them or be absolute—I watch porn and spend too much time on TikTok, too. By analyzing screen time, we free up eight to twelve hours a week. From now on, they'll agree to spend thirty minutes a day, not two hours, on TikTok. Two hours a week watching porn are reduced to forty-five minutes, and six-plus hours spent on Reddit, Discord, Coinbase, Robinhood are distilled to two.

Move It

Many young men don't take advantage of their muscle mass, bone structure, and testosterone to get physically strong. From now on, they'll work out three, later four, times a week—we download an app to track progress. The goal is to start small and build up.

Get to Work . . .

These days, anyone with a phone and a driver's license can make money driving for Lyft or doing chores on Taskrabbit. If you want to make money, you first need to start earning some via a part-time job. A nice thing about making money is that you start developing a taste for it—think Dracula and blood. Money, you realize, is fun and interesting, and making it is a good feeling. Why not see if you can make more? If you work at CVS, do you have the skills and organization to get a job at Whole Foods and earn even more money?

Along with fitness and work, I also ask young men to place themselves in an unfamiliar situation in the company of strangers three times a week in the agency of something bigger—a writing or cooking class, a nonprofit, church, a sports league. The only rule is that within the month they have to introduce themselves to everyone there. Starting with hello, then asking a stranger out for coffee. The other person might say no. The next day, they have to call and tell me how they feel. It might hurt, but guess what? They're not mortally wounded or bankrupt; they're still standing, and that's everything. Now do it again until they start developing a callus. The more nos they get, the more they can calibrate what works and what doesn't. The key, the skill, the talent, the mastery, the ninja artisanship no one teaches, is that the greatest, most specific skill a young man can develop is his willingness to endure rejection.

The above works for most young men; others need more of a sounding board. It's freakishly easy to add value to a young man's life. One young man in his twenties told me he planned to move from Washington, DC, to Alaska. Not sure why—I think he saw a special on the Discovery Channel once.

SCOTT: Do you have a job in Alaska?
YOUNG MAN: No.
SCOTT: Friends? Relatives? Any support system?
YOUNG MAN: No, it'll be a fresh start. Wait, I forgot to tell you—my mom was just diagnosed with Parkinson's.
SCOTT: Parkinson's?
YOUNG MAN: I think that's what the doctor said.
SCOTT: Why are you being such an idiot right now? Don't quit your job in DC: you're making a hundred grand a year!
YOUNG MAN: Oh, okay, good point.
SCOTT: Also, it sounds like your mom is really sick. I'll bet she needs you. Is this really the right time to move?
YOUNG MAN: Hadn't thought of that. Probably not.
SCOTT: Here's some more advice. Bank enough money so you have six months of cushion. Take a week off, fly to Alaska, and see if you like it; you might really hate the place. Also, if I were you, I'd get a job there first, before you move. Also, your mom needs you.
YOUNG MAN: Wow. I didn't think of any of this. Thanks, Scott!

A lovely colleague once asked if I'd be willing to mentor her son, a college sophomore, premed. Dan was feeling low because he'd torn his Achilles tendon playing football and was out for the season.

SCOTT: Are you on the fast track to playing in the NFL?
DAN: [*laughs hysterically*]

SCOTT: In that case, everything'll work out. How's college overall?

DAN: Really good. I'm having second thoughts about med school, though.

SCOTT: Stick it out another year. The world won't end if you quit and do something else.

DAN: Okay.

Dan was fine, I told his mom. The Achilles injury was a setback, but college was good, he had strong relationships, went to church, and was in regular touch with family members. As a successful professional, his mom expected him to follow a certain groove, and right now her son wasn't grooving—so what? Parents across the United States would pray for problems like these.

Finally, I remind young men to cut themselves slack and stop being so hard on themselves. Reminded daily of their own perceived physical and financial shortcomings in a numbing, dumbing, deep-pocketed digital ecosystem designed to make them feel like screwups and cultural outsiders while simultaneously persuading them they can have a viable social and work life on their phones—while other voices online whisper that the world is against them thanks to women, trans athletes, and immigrants—their judgment and sense of reality take a beating. Adolescence is hard, the twenties harder, as one's potential begins narrowing, more is at stake, perspective is limited, and any/all career decisions feel dispositive (see above, limited perspective).

One high school senior I met got rejected by his parent's alma mater. It devastated him. I told him he would still go to college, that there are a hundred great schools in America that double as the best hundred schools in the world. He would get into one, move into a dorm, drink too much beer, hang out with his friends, meet and have sex with women, test his limits, and have a thoroughly amazing time. In five years, when he and I caught up, the only thing he'd be upset about would be how upset he once was.

SCAFA

My anger and depression issues started when I was in my thirties, probably passed down from my dad. I've never been clinically diagnosed for depression, never taken an SSRI. In my thirties, though, I began developing grudges against myself and others. I had a hard time moving past things, would get triggered by something trivial, could feel my blood thickening, and I'd feel hollow and down. I still have trouble getting past things, and periods when I feel nothing—my average daily mood doesn't always sync with my privilege and blessings.

It's not one issue or trigger that makes me anxious; it's more about *me*. The nerve fibers of the spinal ganglia penetrate our guts, where they identify pain, pressure, and more. What makes me go dark is less a function of a bad phone call or a shitty investment decision than my own brain and body chemistry. Once, I was on the phone with my sister when she remarked that I always seemed pissed off about something. "I have to be honest," she said. "You have less right to be angry and upset than anyone I know. I mean, look at your life."

She was right, though I'm still a long way from mastering happiness. These days, I pick up the warning signs more easily that I need to pay more attention to myself. If I haven't exercised, the intensity and frustration that builds up in my body and brain are displaced. I get snappish, monosyllabic, and self-absorbed. I start role-playing aggressive situations in my head that never happened, like a face-off with a coworker, a cabdriver, or an unfriendly barista. These simulations are verbal, never physical. The biggest giveaway is I start thinking about the Holocaust.

I realized certain behavioral changes could help snap me out of it. I came up with the terrible mnemonic SCAFA, short for Sweat, Clean eating, Abstinence, Family, and Affection—my five pharmaceuticals.

Sweat and exercise are good for resetting my system. They're the closest thing we humans have to a cheap, indiscriminately available youth serum—and they make me a nicer person, too. Clean eating means I try to eat home-cooked food versus gorging on trans fats or too many over-seasoned restaurant meals. Abstinence means no alcohol or weed—a short ban against whatever hits my pleasure sensors. Finally, I spend time with my family, even if my sons are being awful and demanding, absorbing as much affection as possible from them, my wife, and our dogs. Love my dogs.

> **Note:** *If you feel low, go back to the basics: Sweat, Clean eating, Abstinence, Family, and Affection. Take care of your brain and body and the rest will follow.*

SURPLUS VALUE FOR YOUR BRAIN

The comedian Bill Burr has a riff where he says men are either angry... or fine. They have no problem screaming at the waiter, yelling at their kids or the soccer coach for cutting their kid from the team. Otherwise, most men, as Dorothy Parker said once about Katharine Hepburn in a play, evidently run the gamut of human emotions all the way from A to B. They're fine, and if you don't believe them, they'll get... angry.

This is backed by experience. Ask most men how they're doing and they'll say something along the lines of *Can't complain*. Most have no idea, I'm guessing.

Therapy-speak permeates social media. Everyone's a narcissist, a sociopath, has BPD, and knows their attachment style. At the same time, our culture is unsophisticated—genuinely stupid—about mental health. I've never seen a therapist—this from someone who for sixteen years, from twenty-nine to forty-five, didn't cry once or feel much of anything. I have friends, though, who've gone or who go and have benefited enormously. Men often struggle to admit they need help or to talk about their feelings, seeing it as weakness or that there's too big of a social stigma or therapy's too expensive. For many, the foundational traits of masculinity, including absorbing the blows of others, can blur the line separating being male from silent suffering (or worse). Pride and shame make for a toxic cocktail. It can kill you.

But vulnerability is strength. By expanding the palette of what it means to be human and male (emphasis on human), you also get to show other men what's possible via example. If they don't get it, it's their loss.

Therapist or no therapist, here's some advice: develop a practice of communicating to friends and family members what you're feeling. If someone or something is funny, laugh out loud. If a book or film moves or inspires you, say so; ditto when you feel sad, anxious, frustrated, or need to be alone. Get used to saying "This sucks," or "This makes me nervous," or "I'm so happy." (Note: it's rarely one emotion—more likely several at once.) I'm not advocating vomiting your emotions at every dinner party; I'm just saying it's a good habit to acknowledge and name what you feel, otherwise you're just sleepwalking through life. It's like learning a language. Sharing your upsets and triumphs with others is, for men, a soft power. It not only makes you feel better, you might also get good advice.

Also, when you share with others that you're not doing well, they become invested in you. Once, on a plane, I sat next to a guy who was the biggest manufacturer of appliances in Turkey; he worked with Whirlpool, Amana, companies like that. We liked each other. It was clear he wanted to be friends. Whatever you need, he said, adding that his friend philosophy, and a source of lifelong pride, was never asking for anything ever. "Then you're not a real friend," I said.

I was reminded of the night I told Adam, my closest friend, that I was feeling depressed that my oldest son didn't seem to want to hang out with me. My son and I had just returned from a college tour, eight colleges in six days. Every night after dinner he went to his room, probably to text his friends. "It really hurt my feelings," I told Adam. "I wish he liked me more." "Get used to it," Adam said. "It wouldn't matter if you were Tom Cruise." He added, "The nice thing is that they come back to you." Hearing Adam, who's raised three great kids, say that, just talking about it, made me feel so much better.

> **Note:** *Develop a practice of communicating to friends and family members what you're feeling when you're feeling it. You're male, also human. Lean into your emotions. Otherwise, you're just sleepwalking through life.*

LET IT BE

From B-school to the age of forty, I was hypervigilant for any time I might have been wronged. The earth would twist away from its axis if I let anyone get away with anything. Every injustice had to be righted, every douchebag needed to pay the price if I, a baller, a fucking *entrepreneur*, wasn't being given proper respect.

I wasn't mean—I just didn't hold myself to the same standards I expected others to follow. If strangers were rude or disrespectful to me, I'd throw it back in their faces. If I was cut off in traffic, I'd cut *them* off. (If I really disagreed with what they did, would I be doing it back to them?) Having worked as a waiter, I had the perfectly sane expectation that anyone serving my table should be impeccable, a mind reader. In the companies I led, I assumed everyone wanted to be like me: awesome and rich. And because I was the leader, they would hang on my every word if only to absorb my messianic *pensées*. Then it dawned on me: *Not everyone wants to be you, Scott.* This wasn't a one-man show where one person gets all the accolades and recognition. The world didn't spin mesmerically around the fulcrum of me.

In sum, until my forties, I wasn't really a man. I approached everything like a corporation: a company's job is to take in resources, add value to them, and get more in return from those resources than they cost. As CEO, I needed to get a deal on everything: *You need to build my website for $30K, not your standard $50K, even if I have the $50K.* But I wasn't a fucking company; I was a person who wasn't winning at all. *How do I get more than what I'm putting out?* I'd find myself trapped in this loop. Some men never escape this mindset. They always have the tape measure in their head: *Am I getting more than I'm giving? Am I getting screwed over?* Then I stopped. I didn't want to live like that anymore. I put away the tape measure. I stopped measuring how I was being treated, quit looking for ways I might be disrespected, started giving people the benefit of the doubt. Basically, I rose above myself. I began giving back. I overpaid people, overtipped waitstaff, realized it was okay to be a better person, friend, neighbor, son, and father than what I might get in return. It was a code to live by—I still do.

SPEAKING OF CODES...

Historically, religion offers a code (or codes): Don't eat pork, don't sleep with your neighbor's spouse, turn the other cheek. The armed services also have one: Never surrender. If I'm captured, I'll resist by all means available and keep faith with my fellow prisoners. Without a code, humans, men especially, can become feral and disorganized. Every man needs an inner structure, whether it comes from family, education, the Marines, church, Buddhism, stoicism, or whatever. Codes don't show up organically, either—you have to develop one.

A code is just a series of adjectives or behaviors that guide and define a person's behavior. With any code, it's more important to be consistent than right. Gentleness and caring, for example, serve as a guide for making everyday decisions. Are you modeling what Gandhi might do, or Atticus Finch, or Barack Obama? My own code showed up later in life. I was always surrounded by men who were good people, but I wasn't able to articulate or internalize or adopt what made them good. Eventually it soaked in. To this day, I try to be three things. The first is generous: someone who gives more than he takes without any reciprocal expectation; second, a really good dad; third, patriotic. Generous, good dad, a patriot—that's my code. I'm not perfect, I still struggle; I'm not some great guy who hangs out all day with his sons, talking shit and roughhousing. I get impatient, I have outsized reactions, I catastrophize things, I talk more than I listen, I get in my sons' faces, I even intimidate them physically sometimes. Without giving the subject thought, writing it down, and committing to being a great dad, I'm not sure it would have worked out as well as it has. Note: if you get angry at your kids, or blame them for something that has more to do with your own bad mood, apologize sincerely. Take responsibility. Acknowledge their (scared or hurt) feelings. Doing so teaches them responsibility, builds trust, and makes the parent-kid relationship more real.

A code matters. If the woman behind the airline counter is hateful, you don't need to be hateful back; she's probably having a bad day—so let it go. If the waiter doesn't bring out your omelet at the same time as the other meals, you'll be fine, no need for reparative justice. Yes, there's a line between taking shit, absorbing blows, and being a doormat. Every man needs to find that balance. For boys, it's important to counterpunch, so to speak; i.e., to test limits via intellect, humor, and sometimes brawn. To know that if you're being treated poorly you have tools at your disposal you can respond with. As you get older, it should start going the other way. An eight-year-old bully is a pill but understandable. A forty-eight-year-old bully is pathetic and unforgivable. The more power, strength, and blessings you accrue, the less necessary it is to punch back against the world. Let things bounce off; most if not all are meaningless.

> **Note:** *Every man needs to develop a code, a series of adjectives or behaviors that guide and define his everyday behavior.*

CHEECH, CHONG & SCOTT

I love getting high. I have dialed back alcohol, and I do edibles now. Two to three times weekly to help with sleep. Basically, I want to run at 80 to 90 percent while giving in to a lot of guilty pleasures. What is the Old Navy of substance abuses?

About weed, we don't know much. Anyone over fifty who's recently ingested a gummy or sucked on a vape knows that this isn't Grateful Dead weed; it's closer to psychedelics. Many cannabis dispensaries resemble Apple Stores—modern, buzzing, nerdy-hip. But ingest too much and your brain turns into a bad Salvador Dalí painting.

There are studies that high-potency THC correlates with and exacerbates serious mental health issues, including psychosis, in some individuals. Low amounts of THC generally reduce anxiety; higher doses can bring on paranoia and panic attacks. Adolescents are especially susceptible, as weed can affect cognition, memory, and executive function. Glad I didn't get into it as a kid, so my brain could ripen relatively normally.

Sourcing matters. Know what you're getting and its reliable effects, or you may find yourself wishing you were dead. Sleep aid? It works for me, though it can interfere with REM sleep, when neuroplasticity and vivid dreams occur. THC accompanied by high levels of CBD helps with sleep; too little CBD and a surfeit of THC can lead to sleep disturbances, insomnia, and feeling crappy when you wake up. Again, if your life is in order and you know what you're doing, go for it. Will it make you "better" at anything? Will it "optimize" you? Will your memory sharpen to a fine pencil point? Will you retain more? Doubtful.

Last year, I went to an event called Summit at Sea. It was on a cruise ship. All around me were high-performing young people who worked in high tech. When I ordered a beer, the bartender said, "Jesus Christ, someone's finally ordering a drink." Wasn't sure what he meant. But in no time, someone offered me mushroom chocolates. This seemed to be how aspirational young people get high. I couldn't figure it out. Wait—I was supposed to nurse a drink while simultaneously doing mushroom chocolates? Was there any upside to this? Or was it just a bunch of wealthy kids trying to show their bald elder that they had found something better?

It's part of a trend away from alcohol, perceived by the younger digital crowd as tired tech. In some senses, this is healthy. Clinical trial data for psilocybin is tentative, but the jury is out. Best to work with a clinician. It's not yet passed FDA approval; ditto for ecstasy. Microdosing on mushrooms just activates a serotonin receptor that leads to more communication—it very likely enhances the capacity for neural plasticity.

ENEMIES OF YOUNG MEN: ADDICTIONS

Addiction is defined as the inability to stop consuming a chemical or pursuing an activity even though it's causing harm. Most people, if they're honest, struggle with some degree of addiction in their lives, including me. It's about identifying and managing it. I like to drink and have been on a journey with my use of it. I'm not physically addicted. Psychologically addicted? Maybe. The closest I've come to needing alcohol to cope is when I started having panic attacks when I spoke. A couple of times, including when I went on *Real Time with Bill Maher*, I would shotgun a beer in the dressing room. Not to get drunk, just to sand the edges. Later, when I thought about it, it sounded a lot like early-stage alcoholism, when you need a substance to get through the afternoon. I've cut way back.

What I am addicted to is the affirmation of strangers. I care too much about what people think. Why would I give a fuck about a stranger's opinion of me? It has no impact on my life. It's the definition of irrelevant. Two-thirds of the really ugly comments I get, the ones that upset me, are from Russian bots, not even real people. They still upset me. Then I remind myself that time is passing, and everyone I know will be dead soon, including me. That's my way of coping with our innate negativity bias and getting perspective, as I still can't wrap my head around AI's capacity to generate a bitchy remark.

Most disease and hardship for our species has been a function of scarcity—too little salt, sugar, fat, approval, safety, opportunities to mate. As a result, when we find these things, our brain produces the ultimate reward, the pleasure hormone dopamine. This makes sense. Nature rewards behaviors that ensure the propagation of the species. But dopa hits then drive our behavior.

Pundits talk about the "attention economy," but "attention" is a metric for addictive products and substances. Our addiction economy comprises media, tech, alcohol, tobacco, weed, gaming, and pharma. Eight of the world's most valuable businesses turn dopa into attention or make picks and shovels for these dopa merchants. The world's most valuable resource isn't data, oil, or rare earth metals; it's dopa; e.g., the fuel of the addiction economy, which runs the most valuable companies in history. Addiction has always been a component of capitalism: nothing rivals the power of craving to manufacture demand and support irrational margins. And in an addiction economy, who is most susceptible to getting hooked? Boys and young men.

Men are more likely than women to engage in all types of illicit drug use. They use alcohol and drugs to cope starting earlier on. They're more prone than women are to excessive drinking, which is linked to car accidents, hospitalization, and mortality. Two-thirds of all opioid-related overdose deaths are men. Twenty million Americans struggle with or are at high risk of developing an online gambling problem. Gambling addiction in men, who are more sports-mad and less risk-averse, is up to twice as prevalent as among women, with suicide rates among problem gamblers fifteen times higher than non-gamblers. Sports gambling is now legal in thirty-eight U.S. states, and, within a year, bankruptcies in many of those states went up 28 percent. In 2024, 72 percent of sports bettors in the United States were male. The cocktail of addiction and dopamine is too much to resist, especially for a group whose prefrontal cortices are still growing. More gamblers of any age can get in deep, fast, and no one will be the wiser. With a meth addiction, your teeth fall out, your skin gets sores. But online gamblers can get in deep and fast in private, with no one knowing.

Today's weapons of addiction aren't just sports gambling and booze and drugs but also day trading, social media, video games, processed fast food, phones and tablets, the bullets provided by social media firms headed by fucked up men-children, the goal being to create in us a simulacrum of their own probably wretched boyhoods. As my NYU colleague Jonathan Haidt put it, the unconstrained combination of phones and social media has been "the largest uncontrolled experiment humanity has ever performed on its own children."

So far, the results are a mental health crisis: 8 percent of teens are addicted to alcohol or drugs; 24 percent are addicted to social media. The suicide rate among teens and young adults has increased 56 percent in a decade. Teens who are on social media for more than three hours a day are twice as likely to be anxious or depressed than those who are on for less than an hour. Is it any wonder Tim Cook doesn't want his nephew on social media? If he wasn't Tim Cook, would he also say, *I don't want him to have an iPad, either?*

By providing real-time dopa for young people, today's technologies implant a persistent craving for *more*—making young people more prone to future addiction. Again, boys are especially susceptible. Twelve percent of boys and men over the age of twelve have a substance abuse disorder, as opposed to 6.5 percent of women and girls. And about one in ten children who play video games show signs of addiction, and 50 percent of all teenagers feel addicted to their mobile devices. Fast food also triggers dopa releases; a third of kids eat fast food every day.

It took us twenty years to wake up to the danger of opiates,

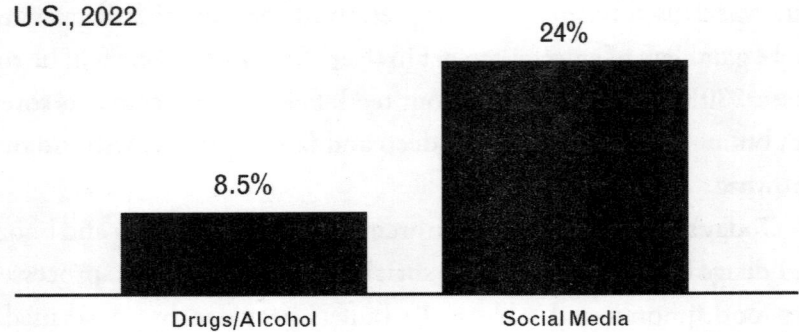

Adolescent Addictions
U.S., 2022

Drugs/Alcohol 8.5%
Social Media 24%

Source: Nuray Caner, Yağmur Sezer Efe, and Öznur Başdaş, "The Contribution of Social Media Addiction to Adolescent LIFE: Social Appearance Anxiety," *Current Psychology* 41, no. 12 (2002): 8424–33.

and about the same for the phone. But it is happening. At least twenty-five states have passed laws restricting the use of phones in school, and roughly three-quarters of schools have policies restricting their use in the classroom. Yondr, a firm that makes locking pouches for phones, has increased sales to schools times ten since 2021, to $2.1 million.

The bulk of the pressure to protect kids from device addiction falls on parents—limiting use (severely) and getting other parents at school to limit use as well so kids don't feel they're an exception. It's difficult, and it needs to be done. An "electronics fast," perhaps for the whole family, can allow the nervous system to reset. Lowering your dopamine threshold allows a smaller amount of pleasure to be satisfying. Try emphasizing, as I do with my sons, the benefits of slow-dopa, where satisfactions are meted out over time. Work hard, study hard, practice, go to the gym every day—and in two months you'll see a payoff.

Congress has been historically lame regarding technology regulation, but when it comes to regulating social media, inaction is par. In the late 1990s, before tech had a major presence in DC, Congress established limits on online services to children under thirteen and the distribution of potentially harmful content. Those days are gone.

Since 2017, Congress has held forty hearings on children and social media and passed nothing. Democrats and Republicans have introduced legislation, including to age-gate social media and to reform Section 230 (which immunizes internet platforms from most litigation), but nothing gets done. Senator Dick Durbin had it right: "The tech industry alone is not to blame for the situation we're in. Those of us in Congress need to look in the mirror."

Richard Reeves recently published a report showing that deaths of despair—people who die by gun, opioids, alcohol, suicide—have skyrocketed since 2004, especially among Black and indigenous Americans. Men today have a higher mortality rate than women in thirteen of the fifteen leading causes of death. Boys and men are four times more likely to take their own lives than girls and women. We will continue to lose more and more and more so long as the greatest shareholder value increase in history is putting fucking Tim Cook and Mark Zuckerberg outside junior high school with a bag of smack. Can you name any substance, any activity, that has a one-in-four addict rate? Maybe nicotine or cigarettes? If you were to say, *How can you really fuck up America?* . . . well, can we do something that makes people addicted, that polarizes them, makes them more prone to conspiracy theories and self-harm? Also, who would we target if we were truly mendacious

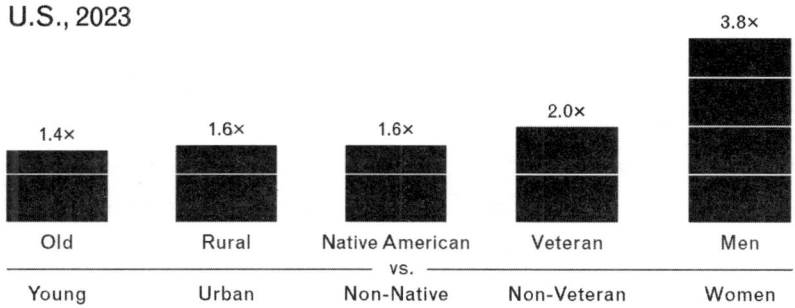

Select Comparisons of Suicide Rates
U.S., 2023

Old vs. Young	Rural vs. Urban	Native American vs. Non-Native	Veteran vs. Non-Veteran	Men vs. Women
1.4×	1.6×	1.6×	2.0×	3.8×

Source: Centers for Disease Control data analyzed by American Institute for Boys and Men.

and evil? I know: thirteen-to-seventeen-year-olds! To set up their brains for addiction and massive needs for dopa hits. A quarter of America's youth is addicted. Meta's stock has gone up. Apple is worth $3.4 trillion. There's money to be made.

DRESSING AND DANCING

Many men don't know how to dress. They walk around with a greatest hits clothing collection, half-batboy, half-adolescent, half-something-they-saw-in-a-catalog. An obvious solution is to get a woman or a fashionable friend involved (moms and sisters count, too). This may all sound sexist, especially what I'm about to say: men are hunters. We're good (or shitty) at making fast decisions, taking risks, inclining to action. Hunters aren't always great dressers. Women by contrast are gatherers. Details matter to them. Their filters are finer. Why wouldn't any man lean into those strengths? Men just need to look acceptable—khakis, a belt, a Gap T-shirt, a V-neck Banana Republic sweater, New Balance sneakers. If this feels insurmountable, do what I do: adopt a uniform so you don't have to think about it.

If an ideal quality for a man is that he be acceptable at a dance and invaluable in a shipwreck, I think the shipwreck part comes easily to most men. This leaves being acceptable at a dance. One of my roles as a father is to teach my sons how to dance. If they learn to move well, I tell them, more women will want to kiss them. This was met at first with excruciating silence: my sons had no interest in dancing with me. I put on fun rock 'n' roll music from my era, which they hate (because they have no taste), but soon they ask if they can take control of Spotify. Sure, I say . . . but only if they dance with me. They put on Kendrick Lamar.

Since then they've come around, or I've ground them down. From TikTok videos, they know how impressive a good male dancer can be. Their schools have formals; they have the smallest glimmer that dancing is a sidelong form of mating. A young man who moves well signals he's bold, graceful, and confident enough to engage in an activity that risks being greeted with riotous laughter.

Why are women often into male risk-takers? They're more likely to protect the tribe. One good way of demonstrating this is via your willingness to dance.

> **Note:** *Dancing is sex but with clothes, shoes, and music—a critical skill for boys and young men to master.*

ENEMIES OF YOUNG MEN: COMPLAINING

Last year my family and I spent some time in the Cotswolds in the British countryside an hour or two outside London. Small villages, sheep on the hillsides—it's extremely pretty there. I reserved two suites in a fancy hotel, one for my wife and me, the second for our two boys. I paid extra so the dogs could come along. There was no reason for me to feel anything but fortunate.

After a late work night, I finally got to bed to find my fourteen-year-old lying next to his mom. He was feuding with his brother and had concluded they couldn't share the same room. This annoyed me. I couldn't even turn on the lights—it would have woken up my wife. After a hissed exchange, the trespasser trundled back to his room, and I got under the covers. I couldn't sleep, dozed instead. The dogs stirred across the room, waking me up. I lay there in the sylvan darkness, pissed off. I fell back asleep. My wife soon got up to let the dogs out, which woke me up again.

The next day, I was the worst possible version of myself, which is saying a lot. I spent all morning complaining about my lack of sleep in my extravagant suite in one of the loveliest areas in the UK. It was so unattractive and unproductive. Was this what economic security brings—a series of lower bars for me to express displeasure and crankiness and feel put out about? The fact I couldn't get over myself made it worse.

One way I know I'm going dark is I start complaining. Complain enough about your life, your job, your partner, your kids, your house, your pets, your car, and you'll become a less viable and productive human being. You'll start to buy your own story. Believing you're oppressed, that you've been dealt a bad hand, that your social/economic background or work experience is positively shitty, that you'll never succeed at anything you do, is paralyzing. Believe you lack agency, and the world and everyone around you becomes your enemy.

Boys grow up expecting to be physically strong, capable of taking on any challenge. Mental strength matters just as much. I've always been drawn to the notion that action absorbs anxiety. Whenever you feel low, defeated, or frustrated, the best solution is to take action. Complaining is reactive; it wrecks momentum. Action restores agency, defeats inertia and self-criticism, and is always available.

At the end of the year, I come out with predictions about business, tech, culture, and politics for the next twelve months. I've had wins along with misses. When I'm wrong, I don't berate myself; there's no point. I learn from my mistakes, but as long as I keep moving and putting in the work, what's the worst that can happen? Most people, me included, are fatally self-absorbed. If I get a prediction wrong, readers might think, *Scott's an idiot*, and they'll go back to thinking about their kids' braces or what's for dinner.

Short of incarceration or online cancellation, our economy and culture rarely penalize or erase people for making mistakes. No one exiles you for a business failure or for being stupid. Here's a secret: Americans love to forgive. We don't embrace failure, but we tolerate it. If you're biased toward action and risk-taking, if you were ready and fired and missed your target, you still get props for showing up and trying.

Action doesn't just absorb anxiety; in an attention economy it also captures and monetizes attention. VCs call this a "growth mindset" (whatever the fuck that is). I call it an action orientation. You may be a member of a historically oppressed group. At the same time, you have more agency living in the West today than anyone in the history of the world.

Young people, young men especially, need to reorient themselves more toward ready, fire, aim (you read that right). In other words, they should stop playing it safe and try on as many incarnations of themselves as possible. Above all, act. Mistakes, pivots, and twists are all stops along the way.

That also goes for mates. If you lack confidence or are risk averse, I guarantee your selection set will narrow. You could very well end up not with a bad person but with the wrong person. As a man, your job is to be a good protector-procreator-provider and build a nice life together with a partner, with or without kids. Use your initiative, perseverance, and risk-taking to approach the broadest possible range of potential mates and remain open-minded. As with jobs, it's less about finding the best one than it is finding the right match. I don't care how much of a baller you are—pick wrong, and it will take ten years out of your life.

> **Note:** *Whenever you feel low, defeated, or frustrated, the best solution is taking action. Believing you're a victim does nothing but destroy agency and make you less likely to take action.*

chapter 6

FRIENDSHIP

HELLO, OLD FRIEND

I've known my closest friend, Adam, since we were eight or nine. On my first day at Fairburn Elementary, a kid (Adam) threw a Frisbee he wasn't supposed to have; it flew away from him, and he climbed a fence he wasn't supposed to climb to retrieve it. On the trip back with the Wham-O disc of joy, he fell off the fence and lay writhing on the ground until the field monitor came over and tried to help. Adam karate-chopped him. Our teacher, observing that I was shy and well behaved, strategically sat me next to Adam, thinking I'd be a balm. Osmosis occurred, but in the wrong direction. In no time, we were breaking into the school on weekends, throwing water balloons at cars from his roof, and leaving brown bags of dog shit on doorsteps after setting them ablaze. Good times.

Karate-chopping aside, Adam had an innate kindness. He was cooler and more popular than me, a sharp dresser, but always included me despite the hit to his brand. For my sixteenth birthday, my dad gave me an old Volkswagen Rabbit. Adam showed up at school in a leather jacket behind the wheel of an Austin-Healey Mark IV. It was like knowing James Bond when he was a teenager. Adam was a bit of a rebel, too. He did drugs before anyone else. Yet he always had that sweetness, and kindness, even after his parents transferred him to a bougie private school. I remember in my senior year I couldn't find anyone to take to the prom. Can't tell you why—at six-two, 135 pounds, with terrible acne, I looked like a construction crane with bad skin. I decided I wasn't going. Adam surveyed the members of his class and found someone for me to go with. That kindness, always.

Our freshman year in college, Adam at Berkeley, me at UCLA, I went north for a visit. I called Adam from LAX to let him know when I was landing. Before hanging up he said, "I can't wait to see you." This may seem trivial, but eighteen-year-old boys in 1982 didn't speak to each other that way.

Forty years later, Adam is still that cocktail of cool and kind. Unlike Adam, I am not an innately kind person. But it would be impossible to be around such an impressive person and not want to model and adopt this feature. I'm a better man because of a boy who used to karate-chop field monitors. A better man thanks to all my friends.

ONLY CONNECT. REPEAT.

Friendship is prevalent across hundreds of species, from chimps to elephants to flamingos. In other words, we are not an evolutionary anomaly. The cynical theory of friendship is that it's a matter of reciprocity, a transaction. Vampire bats regurgitate food and share it with unrelated bats—but only according to a carefully calibrated algorithm based on the other bat's history of sharing its own food. Friends are much more than this.

As I've gotten better known, developed a deeper footprint, I feel I have to do image upkeep: make, if possible, a good impression on people, then exit. It's my imposter syndrome thing. With real friends, I don't feel that way. They know my flaws, my backstory, and decided they like me anyway. There's an implicit level of comfort. I never freak out before seeing them, even if it's been a few months, or worry I'll run out of things to say. Men are competitive—but as I get older, my real friends are as happy for my success as I am for theirs. I'm lucky to count a dozen people in my life whom I could ring up at any hour, day or night, who would drop by or meet me for a drink somewhere. I'd do the same for them. After my divorce, I literally materialized on my friend Lee's doorstep and spent a week in his guest room. When I first moved to New York, I didn't own a presentable suit, and Lee lent me the money to buy one and a nice pair of shoes. I wasn't embarrassed to ask him, nor was he embarrassed to call and harass me a few weeks later to repay him. Friends and friendship should be *easy*, especially as loneliness registers an impact on our well-being akin to smoking fifteen cigarettes a day and rivals smoking and alcohol as a cause of early death.

Despite its health benefits and how good it feels to connect with others, friendship is on the decline. Since 1990, the percentage of Americans who report having fewer than three close friends has doubled, from 16 percent to 32 percent. Put another way, twenty million Americans have begun smoking a pack a day. A number of factors inspired this perfect storm of loneliness: Covid; its aftereffects; political polarization; fewer random encounters, as we no longer go to spots like the mall, theater, or office; social media raising a generation of

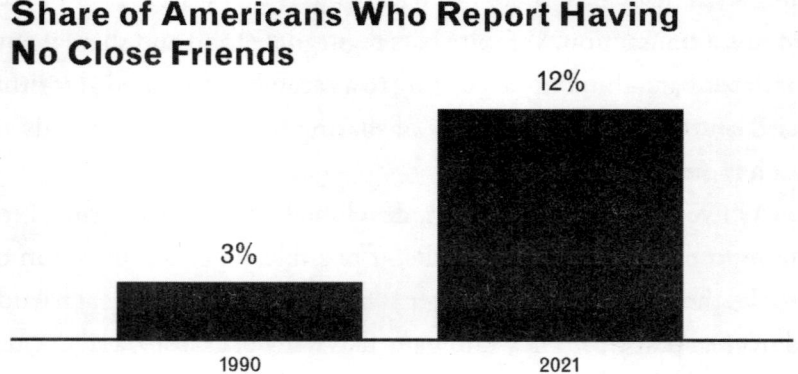

Share of Americans Who Report Having No Close Friends

Source: Daniel A. Cox, "The State of American Friendship: Change, Challenges, and Loss," Survey Center on American Life.

disconnected people who feel shitty about themselves; and a lack of the aforementioned "third spaces."

Men and women approach friendship differently. Men have it drilled into us from an early age that vulnerability and emotional connections are signs of weakness. They aren't. Men with influence have an obligation to cleanse this bullshit version of masculinity from the zeitgeist. The decline in friendship is insidious, as it feeds on itself. Friendship is a muscle that strengthens with use but atrophies with age, but we have to keep pulsing it. We have so many more opportunities and so much more fuel for our friendships when we are children and even as young adults, but we cannot stop building and using these muscles into and throughout adulthood.

Prosperity, distributed inequitably, has made us less happy as many young people turn to online, lower-risk means of chasing dopamine. Young adults' loneliness rates have increased every year since 1976. In the past decade, teen depression rates have increased significantly. As reported by the U.S. surgeon general, loneliness is a national epidemic. It's worse for men, who are stuck in a "friendship recession"—a trend that predates Covid but that has accelerated over the past few years as loneliness levels have increased globally. In a 2021 survey of more than two thousand U.S. men quoted in *The New York Times*, less than half of respondents said they were truly satisfied with their current friendships, while 15 percent reported having no close friends at all—a fivefold increase since 1990. That same survey found that men were less likely than women to rely on their friends for emotional support or to share their personal feelings with them. A 2023 study found that two-thirds of American men believe the statement "No one really knows me well." Who picks up the male friendship slack? Often it's women. Among couples in heterosexual relationships, men rely more on their romantic partners than vice versa. When a relationship ends, male social networks typically contract, whereas women's are unaffected.

Advice: Friendship doesn't happen organically or serendipitously—get out there and be proactive. Practice vulnerability, even if it makes you feel like a klutz. Ignore cultural messages telling you that being emotional means you can't cut it. Compliment your friends. Tell them how much you value what they bring to your life. The struggles young men share are often kept private—you'd be surprised how universal and solvable most are. Be up-front about what's going on with you. If you can't put it into words, maybe your friends can. Put yourself, if possible, in regular social situations over time. Remember that boys and men typically socialize side by side versus the female propensity to interact face-to-face. Don't forget to reach out, check in, shoot off a text or email. According to one 2022 study, casual check-ins among friends and acquaintances are unexpectedly meaningful and profoundly appreciated.

> **Note:** *Having no friends can literally kill you. If that's you, do something about it.*

Friendships offer huge returns. After brunch, working out, writing, or class, walk around with another man you like or grab coffee together. Organize a backyard cookout or beers on the roof. Also, when any positive feeling or thought strikes you, emote about it. Tell

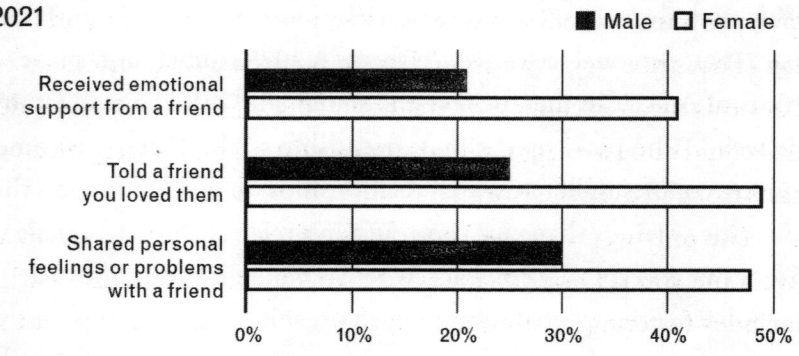

Percentage of Americans Who Report the Following Experiences in the Past Week
2021

Source: Survey Center on American Life.

your friends you hope you'll be friends for life; tell people you are attracted to them, or that they're smart or funny; laugh out loud and touch people (appropriately). We are emotional, physical beings—to not express our emotions in person, through shared experiences, is to be less human. Less alive.

Friendship is also an economic accelerant. The economist Raj Chetty found that for people from lower socioeconomic backgrounds, having wealthier friends "is the single strongest predictor of upward mobility." Unemployed people who volunteer are 27 percent more likely to find work than those who do not, aided by the "social capital" (economist-speak for "friends") they accumulate through volunteering. Regions with greater civic engagement are more resistant to economic slowdowns, and communities to which the residents have a strong emotional attachment see higher rates of GDP growth. The flip side? The CDC estimates that loneliness costs the U.S. economy $406 billion a year—more than the combined GDP of Vermont, Wyoming, Alaska, Montana, South Dakota, and Rhode Island.

Note: *Making friends improves your health and feels good. Friendship can also be an economic accelerant.*

LEAVING THE ISLAND

A million years of evolution have made us comfortable in small groups of other humans, telling stories, challenging one another, and bonding. That's not to say we should make a prison of our instincts. Nor does this mean excluding digital contact. I celebrate that my elderly dad could once see his grandkids on Facetime, and I've recorded podcasts from all over the world.

The only way you will be loved by others, get to love them, and live a life you do not deserve is to take uncomfortable risks—which includes fostering relationships you establish in person. Say yes and be promiscuous when it comes to expressing your regard, interest, and love for others. You will experience disappointment, sore muscles, hangovers, and awkward moments. And, looking back, you will regret none of it. Say yes.

> **Note:** *The only way you will be loved by others, get to love them, and live a life you do not deserve is to take uncomfortable risks.*

It took me a while to learn the importance of friendship in adulthood. When I left business school to start my own firm, I developed proxy father-son relationships with CEOs and CMOs of Fortune 500 firms with whom I worked in my twenties and thirties. The services business is relationship-based, so I would help them get promoted, write their speeches, and prepare their presentations and decks. In exchange they would hire my firm and I would pull together a team of eight people and bill half a million dollars over the next few months. These men trusted me, they were loyal, and I really enjoyed their company. They were what I had as friends at the time besides Adam and Lee.

Then, as RedEnvelope got swept up in the prosperity of the age, culminating in a Nasdaq IPO (the only retail IPO of 2003), I cracked open my life. Blessed with extraordinary good luck, a great partner in Margaret, and the wisdom to be born into the most prosperous era in history, I decided that rather than take stock of these blessings, I wanted more. *More*, goddammit. I wasn't sure what "more" meant... so I opted for different. One day I woke up. I resigned from the board of RedEnvelope, asked Margaret for a divorce, decided I hated San Francisco (the fog, the rapacious businesspeople who screwed you by day and at night, gently candlelit, wrote out a check to Help the Humpbacks), moved to New York City, and joined the faculty of NYU's Stern School of Business.

I had hit a wall. I had built up a slew of expectations around how incredibly successful I was going to be. This seemed to be a habit. I'd even been approached by the Democratic Party about one day running for office in California. I thought I had a legitimate chance of becoming a billionaire. Now I had no obvious career path to speak of. And I started getting angry at myself. Less at the world, and more at myself that I had let myself down.

For the next ten to fifteen years, until my mid-forties, I mostly said no to friendship. I was at home on Scott Island. I made enough money to take care of myself, but had no deep, meaningful relationships, besides a burgeoning relationship with my now wife. I found comfort, convenience, in distance. I didn't have to give or show emotion. I could be—and was—selfish, a mercenary, a solo contractor. I was never disappointed, never expected much from anyone, and vice versa. My crying muscle atrophied. I forgot how. I was isolating myself and I was starting to feel how far I had pushed the world away.

Survival instinct kicked in. While an island nation is a doable strategy in your thirties, it steadily becomes apparent you're making a choice. The choice is . . . death, as men who live alone have much shorter lifespans, and I could sense it. Single men could die eight to seventeen years earlier than their married male friends. Mortality risk is 20 percent higher for those who are socially isolated and 32 percent higher for people who live alone. Studies show the size of a social network—close and extended friends—is linked to good mental health in men. Basically, men with fewer friends experience depression more. Humans are pack animals, and mortality rates, especially among men, skyrocket when we're not actively engaged in other people's lives. Most studies on longevity across genders cite the strongest signal of a long life is how social (engaged) you are in the lives of others, whether it's partners, friends, children, or colleagues. For a fifty-year-old, the biggest predictor of your health at eighty isn't your cholesterol level but the quality of your relationships. One out of seven men doesn't have a single close friend. Reading the Harvard happiness study, they study the checklist: career achievement, check; exercise/good diet, check; close relationships—uh, problem. If this is you, do something about it.

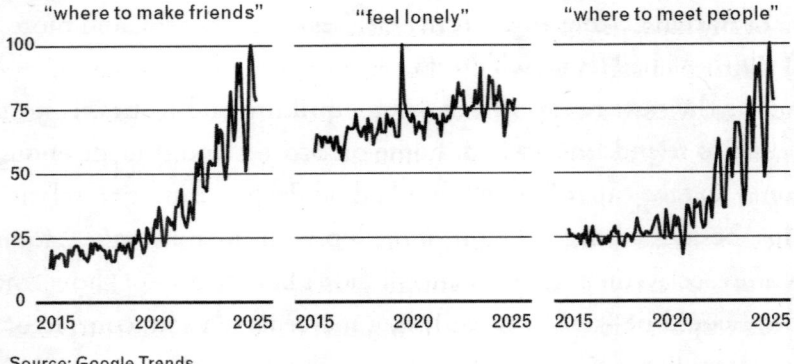

So, in my forties, I realized that if I just had myself and nothing and no one else, I'd remain unengaged and die sooner. Yes, I could continue living my life with no real relationships, leaving my loft only for work, food, and the pursuit of sex. But if I'd kept doing that, I'd be dead now, versus writing this sentence.

THE ROAD BACK

The road back to friendship was fairly cliché. My emotions were there, I just had to learn to identify and speak them. There was no magic moment; it wasn't cinematic—just a recognition, that's all. I thought of aloneness as a physician might. If I were pre-diabetic, I'd stop eating ice cream, and with high blood pressure I'd exercise, meditate, and avoid salt. For isolation, the Rx was and is friendship. It's a medicine I recognized I should take and invest in every day.

As humans, we expect things to be organic—to get on a bike and know how to pedal, to step on a soccer field and know how to kick and score. Never happens. It took practice, incremental improvement. I made an intentional decision to lean into my emotions. Laughing out loud. Crying. Both teach and inform you. The more I leaned into those things, the fitter my emotional fluency. These days, I can't watch *The Last of Us* without becoming a mess. Anytime I talk about my mom or my kids, my voice starts to crack.

I didn't plan on having kids, but having two sons got me off the island, too. Meeting my wife helped me show up and invest in a real partnership where we created a household with laughter, crying, chaos, and engagement.

Let's look at another assumption—that humans are born kind, then start unlearning, or get cynical through experience. Perhaps I was this way as a kid, but I know how much making an effort to compliment people has helped me in the past decade. I lean into admiring others: my partner and kids, my colleagues and friends. With my wife, I tell her as often as possible how hot, wonderful, smart, and great she is and how much I appreciate her (all this is true). A virtuous upward cycle happens—the words lose their mildly rehearsed quality. The more you say them, the more you believe them. Before you know it, you're a better, kinder person. If you envision yourself being a loving, generous person, start being more loving and generous. If you envision being with a loving, generous person or wish your partner were more so, again, start being more loving and generous. It's like practicing to get better at a sport. After a while you don't think about it. What you want is to be someone at ease with expressing your emotions, where you're comfortable with the other person.

> **Note:** *Strive to be at ease with expressing your emotions where there's trust. Compliment others.*

The Iceman still cometh. In moments of crisis or with my kids, it can help to be rational, unemotional—a ballast—sometimes when others are crying, yelling, or flipping out around you. It's a man's job to take the temperature down, to model calm. An overwrought teenager is different from a choleric forty-five-year-old. This is one facet of surplus value—absorbing other people's emotions without taking them on as your own, turning a five-alarm fire into a two-alarm blaze. You have empathy, but you're also the fire chief. Kipling probably said it best: "If you can keep your head when all about you / Are losing theirs and blaming it on you . . . you'll be a Man, my son!"

> **Note:** *One facet of masculinity is to lower the temperature, put out fires, and be comfortable with others expressing big emotions.*

FRIENDSHIP OBSERVED

My mom met her best friend, Karsen Evans, in the secretarial pool of the ITT office in Orange County. Karsen was funny and outgoing and bore a striking resemblance to Amy Adams wearing an Ann-Margret wig. She was a hot number when she was young and derived a lot of confidence from her looks. She married a successful entrepreneur, Charly, who owned a printing business. Karsen and Charly were dear friends to my mom. She even stayed with them after she and my dad split.

In their company, as a nine-year-old, I registered several things for the first time:

- Karsen was the first woman I remember thinking was really "pretty."
- I noticed Karsen and Charly had nicer things than us: a big house overlooking the Valley, German cars, fur coats, and fancy guns from Italy. Karen wore a belt with gold hoops that encased twenty-four ten-dollar Indian gold eagle coins. Karsen and Charly were something I had never encountered or noticed before—they were "rich."

- They also didn't have kids and had fun parties with groovy people who got drunk. They would dance to a live band whose lead singer Charly knew personally. They were "cool."

When I was in high school, Charly would take me to lunch at his firm, and I began to get a sense of work and what it meant to make money. I started to connect work with gold coins and groovy people who listened to live music while overlooking the San Fernando Valley.

Charly was ahead of his time and saw disruption coming and made a bold bet on technology—computers that would replace typesetting. The technology was not practical and required him to change the entire operation of the company at a huge cost. Within two years, his firm of thirty years was out of business, and Charly and Karsen were financially ruined. As with many marriages with financial strains, the strains spelled doom, and Karsen told Charly she was leaving him.

Soon after, Charly was admitted to the hospital with what was then called a nervous breakdown. The term "depression" wasn't yet part of the American vocabulary. After being discharged from the hospital, Charly asked Karsen to go to the grocery store as they were out of Häagen-Dazs. Once she left, Charly went into the garage, put shells in an antique rifle, pressed the muzzle to his chest, and pulled the trigger. Four hundred people came to the funeral—he was loved. I remember the juxtaposition of him taking his life with more than a hundred people crying, his three grown sons (from his first marriage) sobbing uncontrollably, and Karsen wearing thigh-high leather boots, welcoming everyone.

Soon after Charly passed, Karsen had failed back surgery and became addicted to pain pills. She and my mom remained close. When my mom was sick, one day Karsen showed up unexpectedly on the doorstep. She had driven from San Diego to Las Vegas and announced she was there to take care of her best friend. I unloaded her canary-yellow Corvette of its contents:

- Two fake Louis Vuitton bags
- A Maltese dog
- Seven one-liter bottles of Johnnie Walker

Karsen showed up. By then, she was seventy, with big fake boobs. She would help my mom with what I couldn't—showering, changing—when she became really ill. She made Hot Pockets for us every night. I walked in one day and she was naked on the couch with one of the thirtysomething maintenance workers who couldn't speak a word of English (my mom lived on a golf course). Karsen also drank a liter of Johnnie Walker every three to four days. By this math, I figured she had given my mom a month to live, as that's when Karsen would run out of Red Label.

After my mom died, Karsen asked that I look in on her. I called once a month for about six months and then stopped. Too wrapped up in my own shit to call the woman who'd showered my mom when she was dying. So selfish.

I got a call two years later that Karsen had died. She was unable to get a ride to pick up her pain meds, she experienced serious withdrawal, and her heart gave out. Her estate attorney informed me I was the sole beneficiary of her estate (using the term generously). Still, more than I deserved. Just like referred pain, this was love for my mom manifesting somewhere else.

I inherited the belt of gold eagles and decided to keep them in case shit got real—end-of-the-world stuff. I could hitchhike to Idaho and begin trading gold coins for guns, butter, and a few days in someone's underground bunker. You never know.

I hid the belt, a bad idea, as a third of the things I don't hide I lose anyway. I hadn't seen the coins in several years when my close friend Adam asked if I knew there was costume jewelry, a tacky gold belt, in the dresser I had given him. I told him it wasn't costume and that it was likely worth tens of thousands of dollars. Adam said his thirteen-year-old son had been wearing it to seventh grade every day as a necklace, because it made him look like a rapper. He returned it to me.

Karsen and Charly Evans were once the most impressive people we knew, on top of the world, and they both died alone. Karsen was an addict whose only family or friend was my mom. Charly was too sick to register the love from his family. They've helped me see where I've become an addict of sorts, too. Addicted to the affirmation and economic security that comes with professional success. I look at the belt and feel the need to invest in friendships in case they are all I'm left with, and to maintain the perspective that, in the end, all we have is each other, and that's all that matters.

FRIENDSHIP: A PRIMER

The best thing anyone can do to improve their own success is make friends with people of high character who are ambitious. You are the average of your five closest friends. For the past three or four decades, my friends have mostly been men. For a long time earlier in life, women represented two things to me: they could either help make me rich, or I could (maybe) sleep with them. Men could help me out professionally. This was the stupid, closed-minded, transactional, and sexist way I approached my life until well into my forties. No longer. I've spent the past ten years developing really strong friendships with women and am especially close with the women I work with. One female colleague has been with me fifteen years, another twenty-five. I love my male friends for reasons that have nothing to do with me getting ahead.

Your goal at any age is to surround yourself with impressive, good, nice people. As you get older, though, the lanes in which you might feel comfortable narrow. The idea of going on a man-date or investing in a new friendship feels more difficult. The older you get, the more you just want to hang out at home, see your partner and kids, pop a gummy, watch Netflix, and maintain links with the friends you have, without putting effort into new ones.

Socially engaged men face the decision of whether to cap the number of their friendships or not. My advice: Never shut down possibility. Get in the way of chance. I'm always on the lookout for new friends. As we're the average of our five closest friends, wouldn't it make sense that I'd want to keep expanding and upgrading that friend group? The goal isn't to surround myself with doppelgangers; it's more about me learning, getting better, thinking differently. I find friends by pushing the limits. By not being afraid to put myself out there. By going beyond my comfort zone—not just staying home and watching Netflix. By assuming other people are on the lookout for friends, too. Example: George Hahn reads the audio version of my weekly newsletter. During Covid, he came out with a bunch of very funny viral videos. One day I sent him a tweet: *Can we be friends? Sure*, he wrote back. *What are you doing now? Nothing*, I said. *Okay*, said George, *let's grab coffee*. An hour later, we were having brunch in Soho. Recently, the CIO of an investment firm texted me out of nowhere: *I think we'd be great friends*. Think of it as friendship cold-calling. It takes courage and resilience. If others aren't interested, they're not interested. If they bite, you might find yourself having breakfast or lunch with someone great.

These days, in my quest for immortality, I've begun getting PRP—platelet-rich plasma—injections. The doctor draws my blood, spins it in a centrifuge, and re-injects it in my shoulders. It's supposed to relieve aches, pains, and stiffness. I've gone a few times and have gotten friendly with the doc, a young, good-looking guy in his mid-forties. Last visit, I asked him about himself—was he single/married/partnered, gay/straight, did he have kids? Straight, single, and childless, he appreciated my offer to set him up. We began talking about raising boys. Turns out he's the team physician for the New York Rangers. He suggested we go to a hockey game—would my sons be interested?

A decade or two ago, I would have said no. Not his fault. I wouldn't have been confident enough. He was too impressive, and I would have been intimidated. It would have been too important to me to not admit I wanted him to like me and for us to become friends. This happens to a lot of young people in America: for various reasons, their self-esteem gets so battered from hitting roadblock after roadblock while watching others succeed that they give up and foreclose on taking any more risks, whether it's applying for a job or approaching a woman. *Don't bother*, they tell themselves. *You're not worthy; you're not that guy.*

In my thirties and forties, I went to every social event, found the most powerful people in the room, and became their friends or invited them to golf so I could get their business. And for reasons too exotic for me to comprehend, I was struggling with happiness? I said yes to the hockey game. The four of us had a great time.

> **Note:** *You're the average of your five closest friends. Never shut down the opportunity to meet and learn from new people.*

CARE AND MAINTENANCE

Most men aren't especially skilled at friendship (see above). Checking in with your friends might not be the most natural male instinct. I'm good at it. My closest friends and I are in regular contact, usually via text. Last-minute invitations typically work best. Most people plan their lives weeks or months in advance but often have nothing going on tonight or tomorrow. My friends are usually happy to meet up to grab a bite or a drink, spur-of-the-moment. Men aren't complicated—our friendships don't need constant maintenance or oversight. We pick up where we left off, no resentment or hurt feelings, even if we haven't seen each other in a long time. Like texting, male friendships are a long conversation separated by ellipses.

Spending time with those male friends matters to me. So does the occasional all-guy trip. I literally share my calendar with friends and ask them to pick a date and time. If I'm traveling somewhere interesting or exotic to give a speech, I clear out a day before and after and invite them to join me. Four decades after a UCLA frat let me in, I still find great value and joy in male company and collegiality. Everyone in that group has done well in life. Any competitiveness, jealousy, or other petty bullshit has melted away, on their end and mine. It's frankly easy not to resent other people when things have worked out okay for you. One guy in my fraternity group chat, though, seemed to get a heady pleasure from discussing a collective friend who'd lost his job and was having marital problems, until I reminded him of the German loanword *Schadenfreude*. Otherwise, what's left is collective joy at our friendships and adult children to boast about and cap our accomplishments.

As a kid, my mom worked long hours, my dad was gone, and I had no other family around. This may explain why I'm drawn to men with nurturing, caregiving qualities who look out for and take care of me.

CALLING IT QUITS

Some of my friends, like Adam and Lee, I've known forever. Adam I've known since fourth grade, and Lee was a member of my artsy friend group at UCLA, a cadre of cool, stylish, super-interesting guys and girls who wanted nothing to do with the Greek system and would instead invite me to get high and go to the local IMAX or stay in, eat taco salad, and watch *Moonlighting*, versus my frat friends, who were more into drinking beers and singing along loudly to U2 albums before heading to downtown Westwood to see if we could pick up women.

Other friendships I've developed since then can stall or stop. It may sound dickish, but I prune my friends regularly. The ending is either organic or deliberate on my end. One man I was friends with for a dozen years was needy, requiring lots of phone time. In groups, he was responsible for one too many cringe moments—I would end up apologizing for things he said. Basically, I was enjoying his company less and less, not getting much from it, or learning, or improving. It made me wonder why exactly I was in this. Being friends for a dozen years wasn't reason enough to re-up for another dozen.

I'm generous with everything but my time. I'll never tell a friend I've outgrown him, but in some cases it's true (and likely mutual). Make a periodic audit of everything in your life—health, nutrition, exercise, money . . . and friends. Keep tabs on where each area is lacking, or imbalanced, then reallocate your capital accordingly. If you're fortunate enough to be able to spend time with impressive, high-character new people, reapportioning the time you've allotted to these other parts of your life is perfectly okay. So is letting a friendship fade if you're not getting anything—intelligence, kindness, empathy—from it. You can stay friends, and still be there for the people who need you, without scheduling a sit-down and listing off the reasons why your friendship is no longer central.

SOMETHING TO TALK ABOUT

For so much of male history, any expression of male weakness conveyed a signal to other men: *Go ahead, beat the shit out of me, plunder my stuff, take my woman, and on the way out, you might as well kill me, too.* No wonder many men have evolved a discomfort with vulnerability. When men feel vulnerable, their guard goes up; when women feel vulnerable, their guard drops. It explains why some topics of conversation among men are fairer game.

The men I hang out with are mostly comfortable talking and venting about their marriages and kids. With close friends, via sheer probability, I often hear about children who are struggling, though less in a group setting and more one-on-one. Seldom broached are money problems or extremely personal problems like sexual and/or mental health issues. Men typically create a facade around their financial well-being. I get it—men often gain value and status via their economic success, and any concern about their income signals they've fallen short as providers and protectors. But this keeps us from establishing closer ties with one another. As for knottier topics—mental health, sexual problems, or a cocktail—I've never once heard a man tell me he's about to lose his house thanks to a bad investment, that Zoloft makes him feel numb, or that he can no longer perform in bed.

Most men in my experience are hungry for connection and depth, and embarrassed that women are (mostly) easier to talk to than their close male friends, whom they really want deeper relationships with. Try this the next time you're out with a male friend you trust: Go first. Take a risk on a subject that hasn't come up before. Try it out. Note the response. You're seeking permission while getting a sense of what's fair game. This varies. Nine times out of ten, your friend will engage. If he doesn't, no harm done; another friend will. The trick is going first.

> **Note:** *Most boys and men are hungry for connection and deeper conversation. My advice: take a risk, go first, see what happens.*

SHOW UP

The day my mom died, I remember calling Adam to tell him. That night, Adam flew from L.A. to Vegas to spend the weekend with me. We went down to the Strip and got extremely drunk. Adam never asked if I wanted him there, never said, "If there's anything I can do . . . " He showed up.

This reminds me of another friend, Greg. In 2001, after the dot-com explosion, my company, RedEnvelope, went from near-IPO to struggling. We badly needed capital. The company was a monster, too, chewing up $5 million a month. Only $15 million was left, and when that ran out, it was over. The lead VC was willing to invest more but this time based on an exceptionally low valuation. My stake in the company would go from 25 percent to 2.5, meaning the VC firm would end up owning two-thirds of RedEnvelope. Another condition: if I didn't invest, I would have to plow half my remaining shares back into the company or the VC wouldn't proceed.

I was just a founder; I didn't have that kind of money. It was stressful and upsetting going up against a master of the universe VC who'd backed Amazon, Yahoo, and Google. Everyone on the board gave me the coach speech: *Yeah, it must suck, Scott—welcome to the real world.*

I'd known Greg for only two years when he called. He'd heard about what was happening. "Could you use a million bucks?" he asked. "That way, you could invest in your own company and hold on to some of your position." Greg was wealthy, but not outrageously or even close. Parting with a million bucks had to hurt. I said yes. The money showed up in my account the next day. No paperwork, no contract, just Greg sensing what I needed but was too proud to ask for, showing up, and not making a big deal out of it. Note: I paid him back six months later, with interest.

Men have a hard time asking for help. I never told Adam I needed him to come to Las Vegas, take me out, and be with me during one of the toughest moments of my life. I never told Greg how stressed out I was about my company. Neither said, *What can I do? How can I help?* They just did it.

When the Pacific Palisades and Altadena fires of 2025 destroyed seven thousand structures in L.A., I wanted to do more than brood from a distance and send good wishes. So instead of asking my L.A. friends whether there was anything I could do, I asked for their bank wiring instructions and sent them anywhere between $1,000 and $10,000. Yes, pure virtue signaling, but it was genuine, too. When they called the next day, slightly flummoxed, I told them I was coming off a great year and knew how brutal things were in SoCal. "Do me a favor and make me feel good about myself," I said. "Take a break and go to a hotel. If not, give the money to a friend or neighbor or cause who can use it."

This was a big unlock for me, something I wish I'd figured out earlier: a man uses his innate assertiveness to help other people in need... assertively. Wiring money made me feel strong and successful—I was doing what I was supposed to be doing. It felt good. It wasn't a transaction. I expected nothing back.

Don't tell your friends you're there for them—*be* there for them. Don't ask what you can do—*do* it, whether it's dropping off a meal or offering to take their dogs for a few days.

> **Note:** *A man uses his innate assertiveness to help other people in need... assertively. Show up. Don't ask what you can do—just do it.*

CHEERS

Humans have been writing for five thousand years—and drinking longer. Archaeologists recently discovered a thirteen-thousand-year-old beer in a cave near modern-day Haifa, Israel, and there is archaeological evidence of alcohol consumption around the globe by 5000 BCE. Alcohol's draw is a cocktail of biology, psychology, and social norms. Among other things, it lights up the brain's dopamine reward system. For much of history, it was safer to drink something fermented than water—if TikTok had been around before Christ, fitness influencers would likely have encouraged us to drink less water and more Modelo. Through the modern era, we've integrated the firewater into some of our most enduring rituals. Humanity has a deep-rooted affair with fermentation.

But the data suggests that Western culture is undergoing a structural shift away from alcohol as entertainment, social lubricant, self-medicament, or ritual. Everyone but the liquor and hospitality industries views this as a positive development, as alcohol is a leading preventable cause of death in the United States and the number one risk factor for premature death among young people ages twenty-five to forty-nine. Thirty million Americans are in a clinically unsafe relationship with alcohol, and in addition to killing over 178,000 people per year through chronic illness, alcohol leads to nearly sixty thousand acute deaths (drunk driving, overdoses, suicide).

Even light drinking can increase the risk of cancer: alcohol is a Group 1 carcinogen, the highest risk group, which also includes asbestos and tobacco. But we still use it.

Clearly the decline in alcohol consumption is positive overall. Yet it also means a decline in the rites of passage and communal bonding that alcohol historically facilitated (ideally that were done in moderation). It means a decline in drunken hugs and slurred "I love yous," and possibly could result in fewer first dances, first kisses, first dates. Drinking comes with a lot of risk, but it also more easily opens us to new experiences. These don't have to be via substances, but sometimes they help to lower our inhibitions slightly in positive ways.

I've gone through phases with my favored intoxicants: in high school, I hung out with Mormons and did nothing; in college, I drank beer but mostly smoked weed; in my early career, I drank vodka; mid-career was bourbon and rum; and present day, less bourbon and rum and more THC. Intoxicants have been a social and professional tool, as integrated into my life as exercise and eating.

I sometimes feel like a better version of myself a bit fucked up. The very definition of a "good" drunk; i.e., never sloppy or mean or crazy, instead funnier, more affectionate, and more in touch with my emotions. Some fucked-up sense of masculinity still inhibits my ability to express how much friends and colleagues mean to me without a little help inspired by alcohol. Unfortunately, my doctor did the math and told me I had basically been drinking two bottles of Maker's Mark a month, and that couldn't possibly be good for me. So I cut back.

Often, late at night, writing, I'll have a Zacapa and Coke and text people to tell them how much they mean to me. The next day, after reviewing the texts, sometimes I feel embarrassed . . . but no regret. My problem isn't saying things I don't mean when drunk but not saying things I do mean when sober. Hemingway said he drank to make other people more interesting. I drink to make myself more interesting. If the previous sentence sounds a bit pathetic or like a form of alcoholism, trust your instincts.

So it may not come as a surprise the role alcohol played in my male friendships and romantic and sexual courtships. It helped smooth out the awkwardness, dysfunction, and insecurity that can be involved in getting closer to someone. It's a sad indictment, but, scanning my romantic history, I'm not sure I ever kissed anyone for the first time without both of us first having had a drink. While young and drinking isn't always the easiest—or safest—approach to mating, young and sober isn't a walk on the beach, either.

For the past two years, I've been living in London. The UK has formalized pub culture. Like the Premier League, which is 95 percent male, pubs are third places where men (and women) can convene, drink and sing, and let down their hair. Teens ages sixteen to seventeen can order beer, wine, or cider with a meal in a pub if an adult is present. When my oldest son comes home from school on the weekends, we go down to the local pub and order a beer. Our relationship largely consists of me feeding him questions and him offering back one word, two if he's feeling magnanimous. But after a few sips of beer, he loses his epigrammatic cool. He's more emotive and forthcoming. He starts telling stories. We connect. All you want as a dad is for your kid to talk to you. Yes, I get that it's pathetic I must give my kid a drink to have a normal conversation, but it's not like we're doing shots.

Alcohol blurs barriers and sands formalities and self-consciousness. A beer or a glass of wine is an instant commonality shared by friends or romantic partners. Next is discovering what else you share. In a fledgling male friendship, alcohol is a metaphor for lowering your guard. The culture may be souring on inebriation—hey, I get it—but alcohol can enhance connection and intimacy.

Note: *Where the culture, for good reason, sees alcohol and bad health, I still see opportunities for togetherness and possibility when done in moderation.*

COMING HOME

Supposedly each of us has in us bits of every material present at the dawn of the universe. It makes sense—at least when ingesting mushroom chocolates—that our matter will also be present in galaxies, stars, planets, and organisms birthed trillions of years from now. Our stories may or may not make the journey, but the emotions they inspire will become instinct, then DNA, and this matter will disperse. So the question is, distinct from the story you and others tell about yourself, how do you make people feel? When people encounter you, do they feel insecure or inspired? Do you leave people cold or comforted? Do you bring joy, harmony, love?

I'm in a deficit here—I've taken more than I've given. I have a debt to pay. I strive to provide surplus value now. I've started with my boys and am working outward from there. Still time. It's a comforting thought, that bits of us will live on and arrive at distant places trillions of years from now. We all have our longest journey ahead of us. When you get there, when you show up, what will be felt?

LOCAL HERO

This embarrasses me to write about—another story of privilege. Last year, I turned fifty (this means sixty in the Galloway household) and celebrated that doleful fact by throwing a birthday party in the north of Scotland. It took almost two years to plan. I invited forty-five couples, two of whom couldn't make it, and forty-three said yes, meaning there were eighty-six guests in all. Flying to Scotland isn't easy, but friends arrived to great food and Highland Game–type activities, everything from afternoon tea at Balmoral to ax-throwing, because why not? A tailor created bespoke kilt patterns based on how long I'd known each guest; i.e., one for friends from the last decade, a second for twenty-plus-year friendships, a third for thirty to forty years, and the last for people I'd known for fifty-plus years.

Until the age of thirty, I felt ashamed about not having money. As a kid, I remember losing my condo key sometimes and going down to the manager's office for a spare. Inside was a whiteboard where a column read LATE RENT. *Galloway* was always on it.

This drove me not to suffer the same shame in adulthood. From ages thirty to forty, I made just the right amount of money. Later I sold my company, L2, for a windfall, and I now have economic security plus. I'm self-conscious about having this much money. I find online wealth porn obnoxious and wrong. Last year, I went to the WNBA finals and posted some photos online with one word, *Amazing*. "I'm sure it's amazing if you're rich," many people wrote. It bummed me out.

I've never wanted to rub what success I have in anyone's face. I'm transparent about my finances so others can learn from my mistakes and wins and better understand a subject that rich people don't like to talk about. I also know that most sixty-year-old men roughly in my position can't afford to rent a Scottish castle and host their friends. These men are as talented, have the same credentials, and worked just as hard as me. A few twists of fate are all that separates us.

On Saturday night of my birthday celebration, I rose, smoothed my kilt, and spoke for more than an hour. I said a few words about everyone there, what they meant to me, and how grateful I was they'd come all this way.

Warren Buffett tells a story about a Polish woman he once knew. Captured by the Nazis during World War II, she was sent to a camp. She survived, but other family members didn't. Not surprisingly, she had trouble trusting people afterward. Her litmus test whenever she met someone new: *Would they hide me?* That night, I remember thinking everyone in that room would do that, hide me, not because I'm such an exceptional person but more because they're such kind, nurturing, caring people. I've always been drawn to people who are nicer than me. Maybe, osmotically, I've succeeded in soaking up some of that goodness. All I know is that that night, and that weekend, my friends made me feel incredibly loved and taken care of.

I've fucked up a lot of things in my life—relationships, work, balance. But for the past two decades, I've gotten friends and friendships right. My life is profoundly enhanced by the many fun, smart, interesting people whom I've invested and reinvested in along the way, and who invested in me. Hard to imagine a better way to spend money than to have eighty-six good friends crowded into one room to celebrate me while I stand there uncertainly in a kilt, waiting for the ass cancer to show up.

The younger me, who spent every weekend going to cool parties with hot people (or vice versa), cared about only one thing: *Am I having a good time?* If not, I started to drink. I no longer recognize that self. My own happiness today is mostly irrelevant; what matters more is whether my family members and friends are happy. When you're young, you don't spend enough time thinking about other people. At my age, you think about other people more than your own preferences or good time. I no longer have fun unless everyone else is. It's a surplus value thing. Also, progress.

chapter 7

SEX, LOVE, MARRIAGE

THE ENDS

Love and relationship are the ends—everything else is just the means.

When we're young, we take in love—our parents', teachers', caregivers'. When we enter adulthood, we find transactional love; we love others in exchange for something in return—their love, security, or intimacy. Then there's complete love, surrendering to loving someone regardless of whether they love you back, or whether you get anything in return, for that matter. No conditions, no exchange, just a decision to love this person and focus solely on their well-being. Unconditional love has changed my life.

Love received is comforting, love reciprocated is rewarding, and love given completely is eternal. You are immortal. Our role, our job as humans, is to love someone unconditionally. It's the secret sauce cementing the survival of *Homo sapiens*. And to ensure we continue this act, nature made it the most rewarding. To love someone completely is the ultimate accomplishment. It tells the universe you matter, the person you love matters, and you are an agent of survival, evolution, and life. You are still just a blink of an eye, but the blink matters.

Note: *Love is key—it's what matters.*

THE MOST IMPORTANT DECISION YOU'LL EVER MAKE

The most important decision I ever made was having kids—and a happy marriage—with my wife Beata. In fact, the key decision you'll make in life is who you have kids with. Who you marry is meaningful; who you have kids with is profound. (Though I don't believe you need to be married or have children to have a wonderful life.) Raising kids with someone who is kind and competent and who you enjoy being with is a series of joyous moments smothered in comfort and reward. Raising kids with someone you don't like, or who isn't competent, is moments of joy smothered in anxiety and disappointment.

Building a life with someone who loves you, and who you love, near guarantees a life of reward interrupted by moments of pure happiness. Sharing your life with someone who's unstable or has contempt for you is never being able to catch your breath long enough to relax and enjoy your blessings.

Having been married before, and not really ready for it then, I wasn't sure I wanted to again. When I met Beata, my mom was dying of cancer and RedEnvelope had just folded. Not necessarily the "right" time—or a year or two later when she got pregnant unexpectedly. But nothing has changed the trajectory of my life more. And that's almost all I'll tell you about us, because I respect her privacy, so please do, too.

How do you go about finding such a person like I've found? First, override the emotion of scarcity. There's enough love and there are enough partners out there to find someone for you, and vice versa. And that love begins in and with yourself—when you cultivate respect and strength, inside and out, that confidence and love will flow into a relationship. So that when you meet that potential someone(s), you'll have the confidence to like someone who likes you.

And that's my biggest piece of advice when dating: like someone who likes you.

Someone who thinks you're great is a feature . . . not a bug. I've found that most young people don't end up with someone until there has been some form of rejection from the other. Don't fall into the trap of believing someone is better than you because they're not that into you. And if someone thinks you're the bomb, it doesn't mean they're somehow not worthy of you.

> **Note:** *Who you marry is meaningful; who you have kids with is profound. Like, and love, someone who likes, or loves, you just as much in return.*

GUARDRAILS

When I moved to New York from San Francisco in 2000, I lived alone. I had enough money where I didn't need to work hard, and most I could do at home. Twice a week, I went to NYU to teach; otherwise I hunkered down. The density and racket of city life makes introspection a shelter, and I'm a natural introvert. Still, it wasn't a healthy or sustainable life. There was no one to remind me to shower or eat more fruits and veggies or cool it with the microwave. I wasn't unhappy, more that I didn't care about anyone, and no one cared about me. Six or seven years went by like this, the biggest problem being that I had no guardrails.

Men of any age need an organizing principle to help regulate their lives and make them accountable—work, a friend group, hobbies, ideally a romantic relationship. Women typically pour their energy into relationships with their families and friends. They're demonstrably better at maintaining social fabrics in person, too, versus men, who are more likely to adopt a bullshit masculinity template of not needing anyone. Covid didn't help with this.

Loneliness is subjective. It shows up in the gulf between what we hope for and expect versus what we get. The past few decades have seen the U.S. economy growing faster than every other high-income economy, progress seen primarily in gains for the already rich. On other metrics linked to happiness and well-being, America is floundering. Income is stagnant. We have the lowest life expectancy of any wealthy country; also the highest murder rate, the highest number of single-parent families, fatal drug overdoses, and youth depression. And in a lonely culture, social isolation, a.k.a. a widespread absence of guardrails, is on the rise.

My mom was my first guardrail. She always made sure I dressed neatly, kept clean, and had good manners. My UCLA frat was another guardrail, since without the socialization, scrutiny, and camaraderie of my "brothers," I probably wouldn't have made it to graduation. Another guardrail was my college girlfriend. Basically, she told me that if I didn't quit smoking so much weed, she would stop having sex with me. Spoiler alert: this was incredibly motivating. It's now come full circle. My wife will tell our youngest that he's not getting dessert until he finishes his salad. She'll tell me I need to attend my oldest's spring recital; it doesn't matter who I'm interviewing on my podcast. In other words, my fourteen-year-old needs guardrails, and I, somewhat older, still find them incredibly useful.

The positive guardrails young women provide men are formidable. Their presence alone is a positive vote for the overall mental health of a young man. Young men partnered will be fitter, kinder, smell better (they'll shower more), dress better, and be more disciplined and ambitious. Without women around, young men, especially those under the age of twenty-five whose prefrontal cortices are still developing, are prone to making remarkably bad decisions. They detach from the world, put on weight, stop shaving, wear the same clothes, and revert to the same negative surplus value they had as kids.

Human relationships are about connection and compromise, about listening and bouncing off one another in unexpected ways . . . in person. They are about, among many things, the risk inherent in relationships. My advice to young men: populate your life. Get out of the house. Seek out opportunity. Go outward (toward actual people), not inward (Google/Reddit/Discord). If possible, surround yourself with others in the agency of something bigger. Volunteer. Seek out places and people defined by excellence, kindness, intellect, and humor. Find your tribe, your people, whether it's a campus or work or church group, a sorority or fraternity, a nonprofit, a choir, a local club, the armed services. Assume that online dating isn't the best place for you to signal excellence, so be willing to spark conversations with strangers while respecting their boundaries. The good news is you don't have to be in the top 10 percent to find a mate. In-person dating isn't easy and can be time-consuming and expensive, but it's worth it. Guardrails in the form of a relationship can not only save your life, they'll make you a happier person.

> **Note:** *Boys and men need guardrails more than girls and women do. Best is a romantic relationship.*

PASSION, VALUES, MONEY

The best romantic partnerships I know are synced up on three things: passion, values, and money. The couples are physically attracted to each other. Sex and affection establish your relationship as singular and say "I choose you" nonverbally. Every long-term relationship I've had, the woman and I liked and were attracted to each other immediately. I'm not saying this is the right way; it was my way, and worked for me.

However, this is where most young people end their due diligence. You also need to ensure that you align on values like religion, trust, communication, forgiveness, how many kids you want if you want kids, your approaches to raising kids, your proximity to your parents, sacrifices you're willing to make for economic success, and who handles which responsibilities. These things evolve as people do; check in with each other.

Money is an especially important value for alignment, as the number one source of marital acrimony is financial stress. Does your partner's contribution to, approach to, and expectations about money—and how it flows in and out of the household—fit with yours?

> **Note:** *The best romantic partnerships are synced up on three things: passion, values, and money.*

MATING: THE GAME

A key skill set for a young man is figuring out how to approach and talk to a woman while making her feel safe, of course. This requires practice and perseverance, as the line between expressing healthy interest and being a predator/acting creepy can blur, especially when substances are involved. Don't be a predator or act creepy, and instead act with integrity and make sure she always feels safe. Men read about poor male behavior in the media; many fear being defined as exploiters. In my experience, women respond well to men who are straightforward in their interest in them, to men who take the initiative and who know how to listen. They also respond well to men who respect their responses to that straightforwardness and initiative, so long as those men take their time and don't rush things while, again, always, making those women feel safe.

> **Note:** *Men should always strive to make women feel safe.*

TENDER MERCIES

The secret sauce of mating is kindness. Not enough men know this or deploy it. It takes strength to be gentle and kind, as the Smiths lyric goes. One way to show kindness is by expressing interest not just in the woman you're attracted to but in her friends in a friendly way. Good manners—being polite to service staff, talking about your family—help, too. Take time to learn more about who she is, what she likes, what she is excited about. Ask her questions (and listen). In today's bestiary of popular men, masculinity is often conflated with boorishness and cruelty, versus real masculinity, which is kind, protective, and looks out for others.

I recently met a couple at a tech conference. The man was five-foot-seven and Asian. His wife was tall and extremely attractive. Turns out they met at an animal shelter—he rescues dogs. They intersected via kindness. I once saw a study that queried high school kids about who the most popular students in school were, and why. It wasn't the jocks, the grinds, or the beauty queens but the kids who were the kindest, who said, "Great game!" and "You aced that test—you're amazing!"

The fastest way to get someone to like you is to like them first. Everyone values praise and affirmation (from a sincere place) and most of us don't get enough. Why did my mostly Jewish UCLA frat have the highest percentage of women at parties when those women could have hung out instead with the broad-shouldered, handsome Sigma Chi? It wasn't because Jews are known for grad school and making money. No, a few women came right out and said it: *Jewish boys are good to women. They're kind. They're nice to their mothers.* For many women, displays of protection are sexy. This means never taking advantage of another person or putting a woman in an uncomfortable situation. If she's drunk and vulnerable, put a blanket over her shoulders and walk away once you make sure she's okay.

Recently my youngest son told me that a friend, a classmate, had managed to spill soda on his own earbuds and didn't have the $300 it would cost to replace them. My son proposed a deal: If he put in $200—all he had—would I put in the rest? Let's be clear: at fourteen, I didn't give a flying fuck about anybody but me. I would have endlessly ridiculed any kid who spilled soda on his earbuds. (Yes, I was a thoroughly impressive kid.) *We haven't totally fucked him up*, I thought afterward. Followed by *This boy will do well; he'll be successful.* Why? Because he's thinking about others.

Note: *The secret sauce of mating is kindness and consideration of others.*

LAUGHING GAS

The most efficient way of demonstrating intellect without boring a woman to death by lecturing her on Keynesian theory or the history of NASA is with humor. Humor was and still is my social capital for making friends, getting to hang out with people way cooler than me, and, pre-marriage, going on dates I otherwise wouldn't. Basically, I'm funny because four decades ago I was so determined to get laid.

In my broke, single days, I'd approach women all the time. Having no resources, I couldn't flash a Panerai watch, name-drop a recent trip to St. Barts, or flash a nonexistent black Amex card. (These days, owning an iPhone is still a global signal of net worth as it conveys its owner is willing to spend three months of the average Hungarian household's net worth on four inches of glass, copper, aluminum, and tungsten.)

Women often travel in groups—it's easier and safer than going solo. In my unmarried days, I would approach a group of women, say something dazzling like *Where are you guys from?* Next, I told them I was getting a drink and wanted to buy them one, too. (Note: I didn't ask; I just did it.)

You can't make someone be funny—some people just aren't—but humor, the cheesier the better, and leavened with self-deprecation—humor that's so not funny it's funny—works. I used to love talking to women about my investment losses, like *Bought Netflix at $12, sold it at $10, now it's $960.* Laugh aloud, too, and at other people's jokes—laughing is infectious. What made my father not just funny but genuinely hilarious was that when he told a joke, he would laugh uproariously at the punch line. No one understood a word... which made it funnier.

My go-to lines often consisted of bad, corny humor that women, despite themselves, couldn't help but laugh at. Something like *Ladies, do you believe in love at first sight? Or should I walk past you again?* Breathtakingly terrible shit, in other words. But it paid off a lot of the time.

Note: *Being funny is the fastest way to signal intellect—and can overcome countless other perceived shortcomings.*

LIKE A VIRGIN (TRULY)

I didn't have sex with a woman until college. Until then, I was just too immature and insecure to expose myself that way. I spent the ages of sixteen to twenty-five with a hard-on, until I got the opportunity my sophomore year at UCLA. I was also wary—reports were coming out weekly, then daily, about a new plague, AIDS. Beautiful young men with Kaposi's sarcoma were among the walking wounded of L.A., and my friends and I shared a collective nagging neurosis that if we weren't excessively careful, it would come for us, too.

I finally got my first girlfriend. Melanie was super high-character, attractive, and from a wealthy family. It was the first time a woman that impressive had liked and even loved me. If I could wish anything for my sons, it would be to have a good person love them completely early on. Throughout high school and my first year at UCLA, I remember thinking, *I'd be such a great boyfriend. I'm affectionate, I'm nice, I'm thoughtful, I'm funny,* but until Melanie, I frankly couldn't find anyone who wanted to be my girlfriend. Bonus points: she was really into me, and vice versa, and having sex with her was a big deal. It wasn't Melanie's first time, but it was mine. I got us a $29 room at the Bonaventure Hotel, an architectural abomination in downtown L.A., all imposing cylinders—it'll probably be deemed a masterpiece someday if only as the historic setting where I couldn't perform.

Before we went to the hotel, I took Melanie to a play downtown. This was what young men did, wasn't it?—something nice before something dirty. The play ended, and we went back to the Bonaventure. But I was too nervous. I went into the bathroom to put on a condom, but I couldn't secure it; my body refused to cooperate. We fooled around a bit but didn't end up fused. Melanie was fine with it—I shouldn't feel bad, she said. We fell asleep in each other's arms. There I was, with an attractive young woman who liked me, in a hotel overlooking downtown L.A., and my dick had other plans. I thought something was fatally wrong with me.

Practice makes perfect. We were both young and horny enough to try and try again until we got it right, though it took me a while to figure sex out. Physically, meanwhile, I came into my own. Thanks to Accutane and crew, I went from unhandsome to handsome, and sex went from awkward and mortifying to rewarding and fun. If your first few attempts at having sex are clumsy or humiliating and you're not good at it, relax—it's where you're supposed to be. Everything worthwhile in life is effortful. Maybe someday you'll be a young man who falls in love at the prom, the condom slips on like a unitard, the sex is amazing, and you fall asleep in each other's arms while listening to Steely Dan's "Aja" before waking up and doing it all over again. Spoiler alert: most men don't have that experience.

> **Note:** *If your first few attempts at having sex are fumbling, self-conscious, and humiliating, it's where you should be. But the pursuit of sex is healthy, noble, and wonderful.*

ONLINE DATING

Being single takes effort. The prepping, pruning, preening, planning, Tindering, texting, courting, rejecting, Coachella-ing, gaming, and being rejected are exhausting. Being good at being single means you're one of the 1 percent who don't live in the real world and everything just sort of comes to you (I know a few of these people and hate them), or—like any job—you have to work at it.

Studies show that getting married is advantageous economically. Having a partnership, sharing expenses and responsibilities, being able to focus on your careers, and utilizing the wisdom of crowds (couples) generally leads to better decisions (*No, we're not buying a boat*). There is a streamlining of choices, which lets you allocate your attention to things that grow, instead of decline, in value (your career versus your attractiveness to others or being seen at the right places).

Once married, one's household worth grows at an average of 14 percent a year. Married couples, by their fifties, on average have three times the assets of their single peers. Married people live longer and are happier than single people. Higher marriage rates are correlated with greater GDP per capita, greater economic mobility, and a reduction in child poverty by as much as 80 percent. The key? Taking the whole "till death do us part" thing seriously, as divorce seriously eats into the three times the assets. From an evolutionary perspective, monogamous relationships improve survival odds for offspring, benefiting our species overall.

Young men today have fewer venues in which to meet potential romantic partners. With fewer of them going to college or church, and more of them working remotely, men have less social interaction and no ability to build social capital. Those muscles of going out in public, meeting strangers, and going up to women with a fun, funny line can atrophy without practice. And fewer dates and romance means less intimacy, less sex, fewer marriages and kids. Straight young men are often interested in straight young women because they want to have sex. We tend to act as if there's something wrong with that. There isn't. Sex and the pursuit of it leads to romance and intimacy. It lights a fire under young men to better themselves to be more attractive to potential mates, who help them reach their potential. This intimacy often involves sacrifice, the forsaking-all-others stuff that comes when a pair of young people say, *I choose you.* This often leads to children. The most wonderful things in life, in my experience, lack rationality and structure. The person you fall for, and how it happens, will likely make less sense than almost any other important thing in your life. And that's one of the reasons it's so great. It speaks to you on a different level. Not what society or your parents want, but what you do. And, eventually, the answer to the most important question of your life: Who do you want to build a life with and have a family with?

FAMILY MATTERS

Families are the foundational element of society, and most successful families are the product of an intimate relationship between two adults. Except, according to Gallup, only about 21 percent of Americans under thirty have kids. In 1980, the figure was about 38 percent; in 1950, it was around 50 percent. There are many reasons why: a corrosive political ecosystem, worry about climate change, people living longer, and the astronomical expense of raising children all the way through to college.

The path to children typically involves sex. If a young adult hasn't had sex in the past year, it's unlikely that person is on the path toward a long-term bond with someone and subsequent offspring. To be clear, I'm not suggesting that it is any one group's responsibility to sexually "service" another. What we need to be thoughtful about is how our policies and attitudes ensure that the most people have the opportunity and motivation to pursue long-term, productive, healthy relationships.

MEET UP (ONLINE)

We used to meet potential mates at school, at work, through friends, and out in the world. No longer.

Online dating shares flaws with other technologies that scale our instincts. Algorithms are indifferent to social interests, and that, coupled with human nature, gave us January 6 and QAnon.

Dating apps sort potential partners into a tiny group of haves and a titanic group of have-nots. On Hinge, the top 10 percent of men receive nearly 60 percent of the "likes"; the comparable figure for women is 45 percent. The bottom 80 percent of male Tinder users, based on percentage of likes received, are competing for the bottom 22 percent of women. If it were a country, Tinder would be among the most unequal in the world.

What is driving this division? As with so much else online, dating apps don't change human nature; they focus it. Regardless of how we meet potential mates, we sort them in large part based on looks and earning potential. Algorithms magnify that effect.

As dating apps lose popularity for these very reasons, look up and around you when you're out, to see if anyone catches your eye. Talk to strangers. Be open to possibility.

WINNER TAKE MOST

Marriage rates in the United States have been steady for a while now. While the social pressure men and women once felt to get married has loosened, many women no longer have to wed for financial reasons. Only 34 percent of single women were looking for romance, according to a 2022 Pew survey of single adults, compared with 54 percent of single men, a decline from 38 percent and 61 percent just three years earlier. The reasons include an increase in women's economic power, a growing mismatch between male and female educational background and economic prospects, and expectations on the part of men that their wives or partners should give up their professional ambitions in favor of family and domestic life—or do the bulk of the housework and taking care of the kids while working a full-time job while the man focuses mostly on *his* job.

The group that's seen the sharpest decline in getting married?

Poorer men. Between 1970 and 2011, the marriage rate for the lowest-earning quartile fell by nearly 35 percent, while that of the highest quartile fell by less than 15 percent. In the past forty years, coupling has declined more than twice as fast among Americans without a college degree, compared with college graduates.

The most powerful signal of earning potential, especially for people in their twenties who haven't yet realized their potential, is a college degree. College-educated men earn a median $900,000 more over their lifetime than those who only graduated from high school. A college degree also increases your chances of getting married by 30 percent.

Marriage rates among college-educated women have held steady at around 70 percent for decades. The decline in marriage rates has been among women without a BA. As a result, a huge class gap in marriage has opened up. Crunching the math: one in five women with college degrees are marrying men without college degrees, resulting in an increasing number of men in the body of the pyramid who will be left not merely without sex, but also without any on-ramp to the intimate relationships on which so much of their happiness, and our social capital, is built.

SECOND-ORDER EFFECTS

So what? America spent its first three hundred years treating women as second-class citizens; what's wrong with young men finding themselves at an educational disadvantage? (Though women are also hurting in this equation.) If this were just about fairness or feelings, then fine, let there be churn. But there are several externalities that could have profound effects on our commonwealth and the global community.

First, less partnering and propagation means fewer babies. Declining birth rates can have negative impacts on economic health. For a glimpse at the declining-birth-rate future, look at Japan, where birth and marriage rates have fallen to record lows. There are now just 2.1

working-age Japanese for every retiree, the lowest ratio in the world. In the United States there are 3.9. The world average is 7.

Second, a large and growing cohort of bored, lonely, poorly educated men is a malevolent force in any society, especially this one. While violent crime of all kinds is down sharply in recent decades, men are already more prone than women to believe in conspiracy theories. Increased frustration about their lack of life choices and greater jealousy stoked by the images of success they see on their screens will push less educated men further toward conspiracy theories, radicalization, and nihilist politics. Global problems, including climate change and more frequent pandemics, require a massive investment of human capital and a renewed respect for intellectualism—and science.

Third, while the forces of technology and social change are chipping away at on-ramps to intimacy and relationships for young men, it's unlikely they will lose their political power. This may be the dark heart of the matter. Politicians will emerge from this class, and many more will pander to them. Today's blowhards aren't an anomaly—privileged men of wealth rising to power on the message that *this isn't your fault*, and then demonizing other groups, is a greatest hits of nationalism and the fascism it often inspires.

PARTNER

Our partners encourage us to take smart risks, compensate for our weaknesses, and (in a healthy relationship) have the strength to tell us when we're doing something wrong, unfair, or just plain stupid. Good partners protect you from others; great partners protect you from yourself. It's also true on sports teams, boards of directors, and in ensemble movie casts.

Everyone needs counterweights. Indeed, the more weight you carry, the more you need others to balance you. Some of the most valuable advice I get isn't about what to *do* but what *not* to do. The wisdom of crowds (i.e., a small crowd of people who are smart and care about you) will help you make better decisions, or at least ask, *Have I really thought this through?* I've done so many dumb things in my life. Until the age of forty, I defined "leadership" and being a man as assessing a situation quickly, making a decision, and trying to persuade everyone around me I was right. Wrong. The most successful people I know, and meet, have a common trait: they ask good questions—lots. It helps them make better decisions. I didn't figure this out until later in life, and I did so then in large part thanks to my wife.

The best decisions I've made? Mostly avoiding errors of omission, not commission. Without my partner's influence, I would never have had kids, wouldn't have bought our house in Florida, or moved to London, or even gone out to dinner last night. A few fifteen-car pileups have been averted, though, because she, or someone else, said, *Hey, maybe . . . don't.* Or, beneficially, *Do.* For example. I didn't want to invest in Florida real estate, but, thanks to my wife, we did and our house has since quadrupled in value.

Focus on your relationships. Family and friends are essential to long-term happiness, and the most important relationship is with your spouse. Marry the right person and then invest in that relationship every day. Don't keep score, and bring forgiveness, generosity, and engagement to your spouse, yourself, and your marriage. In sum, show up.

> **Note:** *Good partners protect you from others; great partners protect you from yourself.*

SHE'S THE ONE

On the first podcast I was ever on, I made a bunch of stupid jokes about my wife. After, she asked me not to bring her up again. I said I wouldn't. When my editor asked, I told her that the reality is that part of my life—marriage, family—is really good, a huge source of comfort and reward for me. I just don't talk about it. The public aspect of our lives together is one my wife doesn't especially relish—it's a privacy thing. Her absence in this chapter, and the absence of any up-close-and-personal details or further discussion of our marriage, is in no way meant to diminish the most important person in my life. I was incredibly lucky to be given the opportunity to raise two boys with a person I love, and who loves me, and who's a high-quality person with her own impressive career. She and our family are, to me, home, ground zero. Her omission from this chapter is one way I protect her.

I will say this much: it wasn't a Hallmark Channel love affair. There was no snow falling; there were no hand-knit scarves. She wasn't a small-town vet or kindergarten teacher dissolving the defenses of a brash, depressive urbanite with fan belt problems, and I wasn't a hunky snowman come to life, either. We met by the pool at the Raleigh Hotel in Miami. Overhead, a deejay was spinning tunes. It's never easy to go up to a woman under the midday sun without alcohol involved, but I felt I needed to say something to her. My words trickled out, a golden elixir of eloquence to her and her friends: *Where are you guys from?*— my follow-up thought being *I'll bet she'd be fun to hang out with.*

We slowly started hanging out together. For the first three to six months, we would go out, eat, end up at a club, dance, drink too much, go home, fall into bed. No pressure, no commitment—neither of us was serious. We soon realized we enjoyed each other's company a lot. *A lot.* A good reminder that nothing wonderful will ever happen to you unless you take an uncomfortable risk by spending time with people you don't think you're going to marry.

> **Note:** *Spend time with people you don't think you're going to marry. You might be surprised.*

I always assumed I'd marry a Jewish woman, another academic, not a woman lounging poolside. Nor was she expecting to meet a thirty-nine-year-old going through a full-blown midlife crisis. Initial attraction, followed by love and intimacy, and eighteen months later our first son was born. Note the order: attraction came first. Then everything else lined up.

We've been together now for twenty-two years. It's a fantastic partnership. Marriage and family are the most rewarding parts of my life. The best relationships and marriages combine yin and yang; e.g., one person stacks the dishwasher like a Swiss architect, and the other is like a raccoon on meth. We're the architect/raccoon combo. My wife is plainspoken, has a temper, blurts out things, and then it's over, whereas I'm usually quieter but also a mess since I internalize and catastrophize everything.

I'm no marriage expert but here's my advice to young men: find a woman you want to have sex with, be affectionate with, and spend time with. A great marriage is one where you genuinely want the other person to win, where you celebrate and relive each other's victories. You want to be on the same team—and then *are* a team. Whenever anything good happened to me in my twenties and thirties, the first person I called was always my mom. She would revel in my success. Trumpeting my wins to friends felt obnoxious and unseemly (because it was and still is), but I could tell my mom I got a $35K bonus at Morgan Stanley and absorb her pride and happiness. Even now, whenever something good happens, my first instinct is to dial my mom. Since she's not here to celebrate with me, it sometimes feels like the good thing didn't happen.

I do the same with my wife. She texted me recently that she'd had a conversation with our son's teacher, who had commented on how great he was doing in school, and she was excited. I waited until she was home, then called her so the two of us could revel in it. (Then I went back to thinking about myself.)

> **Note:** *Find a woman you want to have sex with, be affectionate with, and spend time with. A great partnership is one where you genuinely want the other person to win, where you celebrate and relive each other's victories.*

PORN-FREE

The most underreported addiction out there is porn. It's understudied, too—there's little to no peer research. Not a ton of academics are eager to claim porn as their domain of expertise or are competing to be known as Professor Porn. Porn addiction isn't listed in the *Diagnostic and Statistical Manual of Mental Disorders* (*DSM*); it's self-diagnosed. There's no blood test or fMRI to confirm you're overdoing it.

I was at a conference in Barcelona last year for the biggest digital firms. A kid who runs a successful cybersecurity company and clears a few million annually asked if I would mentor him. "Boss," I said, "maybe you should mentor me, because it doesn't sound like you're struggling" (these were my exact words). Then he said he was addicted to porn. It was immediately clear he regretted opening his mouth. He's one of a half dozen young men I've met in the past six months who've told me porn is their drug of choice. I suspect they aren't outliers but canaries sounding an alarm from the most opaque sector of the addiction economy.

At the turn of the millennium, there were no social media platforms, there wasn't enough bandwidth to run video, and Amazon was a bookstore. But online porn dates back to 1995. By 2004 online porn was so ubiquitous that *Avenue Q* won three Tony Awards, including Best Musical, with a song called—wait for it—"The Internet Is for Porn." Nobody doubted that claim then, and nobody doubts it now. But how much of today's internet is porn? We're not sure. Some estimates put porn-related traffic as high as one-third of all internet traffic. Pornhub, the leading distributor of free, ad-supported porn, ranks in the top twenty websites globally; ten of its competitors rank in the top one hundred.

Humans came off the savanna hardwired for addiction. The dopamine rush a hunter felt when taking down a mammoth is neurologically the same feeling a gambler gets when betting. Our instinct to gorge whenever we see food was honed during millennia of scarcity, and it's that same instinct the food industrial complex leverages to keep people eating long past the point of being satiated. Companies capitalize on human instincts to maximize profit. The most recent figures for Aylo, the company behind Pornhub, Brazzers, RedTube, YouPorn, and Xtube, showed 2018 revenue of $460 million, with a profit margin of 50 percent. In a study of two thousand adults, 11 percent of men and 3 percent of women reported some agreement with the statement "I am addicted to pornography"—fewer people than report alcohol abuse, but more than admit to a problem with gaming or gambling.

Meanwhile, OnlyFans generated $6.6 billion in revenue in 2023. The firm has more than 300 million registered accounts, of which 70 percent are male. On the other end of that internet connection are 4.1 million creators, 84 percent of them women. During its peak growth, OnlyFans was adding the population of Atlanta to its registered user base every day. While OnlyFans is known for its subscription model, one-off transactions are driving 88 percent of the revenue growth. These "tips" are an arbitrage on the disparity between the biological impulse to mate and the lack of mating opportunities.

While sexbots and AI assistants are inexpensive and don't need vision and dental, they are not real and don't nourish our soul. We're not wired to live in a world where we have friends but don't experience friendship and rely instead on Reddit, Discord, and Google. Similarly, we're not built to connect with personalized videos of women as a substitute for real intimacy, sex, and love.

We are what we pay attention to. More research is needed, but one study found that porn consumption explained 9 percent of the variation in men's sexual objectification of women. Among men who prefer degrading pornography, the variance increased to 20 percent. A longitudinal survey of 962 Dutch adolescents found exposure to porn among males was a strong predictor of objectifying attitudes toward females. Porn, mostly harmless in moderation, becomes, when used in excess, a stealth wrecking ball, disfiguring ambition, romance,

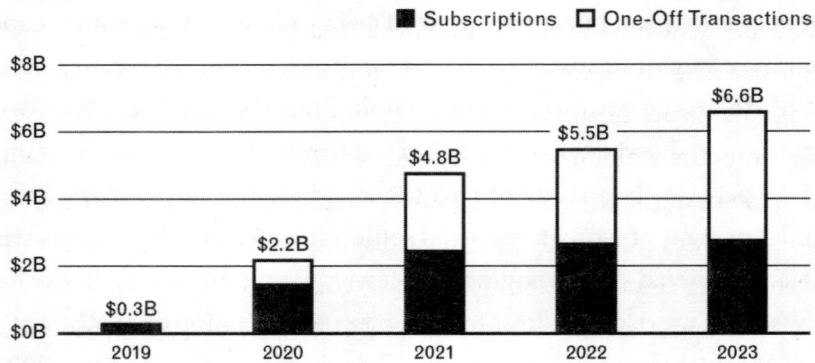

Source: Matthew Ball, "Breaking Down OnlyFans' Stunning Economics," MatthewBall.co, September 8, 2024, https://www.matthewball.co/all/ofpl.

partnership, your attitudes toward women, and your own mental and physical well-being.

If addiction can be defined as doing something that damages other areas of your life, there've been periods of my life when I technically qualified as being addicted to porn. I realize it's unrealistic to tell anyone to abstain from it. Let me be clear: I like porn. I struggle with it, too. I modulate my use and try to be purposeful about it.

If you're alone, bored, anxious, or can't sleep, porn can be a healthy distraction (not sure most women understand the role porn and masturbation play in men's lives). It's fine in moderation, and most men are skilled at jerking off. Too much and you risk objectifying women, preferring a screen to in-person connection, and losing the fire. Don't cut yourself off from the potential, the awkwardness, growth, and magic, that can come via intimacy and sex with actual people.

In college, I majored and minored in horniness. I would leave my room and head over to campus for one reason: to meet and chat up women in the somewhat quixotic hope we might end up having sex. If online porn had been around, I wouldn't have bothered. Horniness is healthy. It inspires young men to take risks, make contact with women, and create opportunity. In the same vein, I made eye contact with my female classmates, our back-and-forths a kind of foreplay. You heading to history class, too? Hey, we're having a frat party on Thursday; you should swing by, bring your friends! Eighty percent of the time, the woman would show up at the party and ignore me, and 20 percent of the time we'd end up fooling around. It made everything worth it. More, it created an upward spiral of me getting comfortable with taking risks and getting to know women.

Mating is hard. I can't even quantify how much rejection I've endured from women. With porn at my disposal, I wouldn't have made the effort. Eliminating or moderating porn use helps young men flex their risk muscles, which has cascading effects on all other areas of their lives. The zillion-dollar skill for young men isn't getting a woman to agree to have coffee; it's about putting yourself in situations where you ask a woman out, she says no, and you realize you're just fine. Eventually you'll get to yes. Watching porn sharply diminishes even the opportunity to get to no.

Also? A key to a successful marriage is reserving and allocating your sexual energy for and toward your wife. Unhealthy dependence on porn quite frankly means you won't be as motivated to have actual sex. I understand—children and work stresses and familiarity can be sex killers. But even if they're not up for it, expressing sexual desire toward them matters to women. Women want to be wanted. There have been times when I was consuming enough porn that it wrecked my mojo and sexual energy for my wife. This is no good.

According to Dr. Anna Lembke, a professor of psychiatry at Stanford, addiction is a disease of loneliness, and all drugs, porn being one, are ersatz replacements for human connection. Instead of connecting, addicts isolate, shelter in place. With their behavior meeting their needs, there's no incentive to seek human company. If porn is in the way of your taking risks, establishing friendships and relationships, building the skills you need to make yourself socially and professionally successful—if it feels out of control and you keep telling yourself you're going to stop but can't—be honest with yourself. Find an individual or group therapist or a twelve-step program (some have virtual meetings). Porn is a masculinity killer. If working out and creatine build you up and make you stronger, porn makes you weaker and less motivated bit by bit. It quashes your mojo for getting out there and creating your own bad porn.

We pathologize males attracted to misogynistic communities as incels, potential mass shooters, and sex criminals, but these men are statistical outliers. However, we may be evolving a new species of asocial, asexual male: *Homo solo*. *Homo solo*'s inability to develop romantic skills means he's primarily a danger to himself, as he's likely to be less happy, earn less money, and die sooner. *Homo solo*'s AI girlfriend never says no and is never tired, busy, or in a bad mood. In other words, she's not human, and that obviates the risk of rejection and the other complexities of real-life relationships.

> **Note:** *Porn is a risk- and masculinity-killer. If working out and creatine make you stronger, porn makes you, bit by bit, weaker. Moderate its use. Get help if it's a problem.*

DEATH AND DIVORCE

The two most impactful things are death and divorce. My parents' divorce was seminal and formative—it shaped the rest of my life. My own divorce was my first big personal failure—a failure of character. She, Margaret, was a wonderful person—salt of the earth, kind, ambitious, and really attractive. We were together from the ages of twenty-three to thirty-five, very much in love, very compatible, and together we built a really nice life. *You scored out of your league, Scott,* people always said. After business school, we got married. We were both working hard. We bought a great house in San Francisco, had great friends, a great life, and were starting to think about kids. It was a good first marriage, probably better than most enduring marriages. Then I blew it.

The honest truth was that on my trips to New York I was exposed to a riotous buffet table of people my age and younger who were doing super-interesting things. The nightlife was intoxicating. I finally had entree to that ecosystem. I was making money, my sexual currency was growing, and I could signal resources. Immature and selfish, I was seduced by a lifestyle I'd never had access to, not just other women but also different sets of experiences and opportunities. Once, on a business trip there, I got invited last-minute to Fashion Week in Milan. I said I was busy that week—kidding, I went. Back at home, it hit me: I wanted to be single and wealthy and living in a New York City loft, partying at Lotus and Pangea, vacationing in St. Barts, and occasionally advising a hedge fund. Maybe that made me a bad person; I don't know. So I did the (again, incredibly selfish) math and concluded I needed to spend the next five to ten years scratching that itch. Basically, I broke a promise.

I knew I couldn't find a better partner. But more than doing better, I wanted to do different. I told Margaret I was struggling with being married. We went to see a marriage counselor. During the first session, I immediately broke into what an impressive woman Margaret was and how much I loved her. Stop, the counselor said. There are two cities, he said. The first is Marrytown. Marrytown—which is, among other things fiscally smart—centers on companionship and its rewards; also security and safety. Living in Marrytown, you get to sleep every night beside a good person you know, trust, and love. Living in Marrytown, though, requires a certain level of commitment and sacrifice. It also features a few ring fences, some of them electric. You give up a measure of freedom—you can't just take off or be 100 percent selfish; you also can't sleep with other women, and your time doesn't always belong to you. The second city is Singletown. It's lonelier, less secure, likely to be filled with stretches of depression and purposelessness, but it promises some unpredictably rewarding moments, too. In Singletown, you can be selfish as hell, do whatever you want whenever you want. "Scott," said the counselor, "imagine Margaret's not in this room. What city do you want to live in, Marrytown or Singletown?"

I'd already decided. "Singletown."

"Then you should get divorced." We didn't have kids, he went on, and we were both making good money. If Singletown was my city of choice, now was as good a time as any to pack and move. Margaret broke down in tears. We left the office. That was the end of our marriage. That day or the next, we sat down together. We listed our combined assets on a yellow legal pad. I offered her 60 percent of everything as a sort of guilt tax. The low-cost New York lawyer I found assured me he could come up with a better deal, but I wasn't interested. I wanted it to be done, over.

There are no profound lessons here except maybe we got married too young. You and the person you marry will be different people ten years from now, which means you'll have to invest effort and generosity in your relationship if you continue growing together. At the time, I lacked that generosity and maturity. Getting divorced was the hardest decision I ever made, but also the smartest. It sounds harsh, but if I'd stayed married, my resentment would have infected everything. I would have become a serial infidel, an unkind, self-absorbed, untrustworthy husband. Margaret was a wonderful person and wife. The look of hurt, shock, dismay, and resignation on her face when I said "Singletown" still makes me shudder to remember. She couldn't fix or improve the situation; i.e., she couldn't change *me*. I don't regret getting divorced, but that moment in the counselor's office is to this day the most I've ever hurt another person. Margaret went on to marry a really nice guy and have a kid. We both ended up better off, and a lot happier, too.

One of the young men I mentor is named Gabriel. He's twenty-one, is doing really well, has a good job and an excellent relationship with his parents. He's also engaged to a nineteen-year-old named Miranda. She's lovely. They're both committed to each other. But when he told me that, it was a big red flag. I told him that thirty-one-year-old Gabriel will be significantly different from twenty-one-year-old Gabriel; ditto for twenty-nine-year-old Miranda looking back at her nineteen-year-old self. "I'm not suggesting you break up," I told Gabriel. "I hope you two grow together." Margaret and I were twenty-two and twenty-three when we met. I was instantly enamored, felt so fortunate to be with her, that when the twenty-seven- and twenty-eight-year-olds in our friend ecosystem began getting married, it felt contagious, even though we were younger.

None of us knows the person we'll be a decade from now. Readiness means different things to different people. At twenty-three, I was "ready" to marry, the problem being I didn't take into account my future self. When I did, finally, in my selfishness I seriously hurt an incredible woman. I'm not proud of that.

THE COSTS OF DIVORCE

While divorce is legally available today, it remains expensive (the median U.S. divorce costs $7,500), and in the short run it's emotionally grueling. Women initiate most divorces (perhaps as many as 70 percent), but they also bear the brunt of the financial impact: women typically see a decline in income for years afterward and have a more difficult time re-partnering. It's even harder for women with children. The data on long-term psychological well-being after divorce is mixed, but men may experience greater emotional harm.

The most profound costs of a split don't fall on the couple. Divorce is hard on kids and the consequences persist into adulthood. Note: kids are almost never "resilient." I remember, at the age of ten, registering that I was a liability in the eyes of the men who'd arrive at our door to take my mom on a date. Children of divorced parents are on average unhappier, more anxious, and more likely to be depressed. They're also less likely to graduate from high school and college, typically make less money, and are more likely to ultimately get divorced themselves. But: *the same is true of children whose parents stayed in a high-conflict marriage.* Relationships that breed severe conflict can be as hard on children as breakups. Chaos is the culprit, not legal status.

Divorce has been at the center of the most disturbing periods in my life: when my mom told me we weren't going home; when I acknowledged my own immense shortcomings after telling my wife I wanted a divorce; and most recently, when I watched my father leave his wife of twenty-five years two years before she died of Parkinson's. Just as Jane Goodall was profoundly disappointed when she realized that chimpanzees are like us, wildly imperfect, divorce brings you face-to-face with your flaws and the collateral damage they levy.

> **Note:** *Children of divorced parents and parents who stay in their high-conflict marriages are on average unhappier, more anxious, more likely to be depressed, and less likely to graduate high school and college.*

CONSCIENTIOUS UNCOUPLING

The liberalization of divorce laws initially freed many couples from unhappiness, literally saving the lives of women shackled to abusive men. But it remains exorbitantly expensive to end a marriage that should end, and our society struggles to provide a stable environment for kids that doesn't rely on having two parents under the same roof.

Undoubtedly, we need better marriages. Do we want fewer divorces? Are the exit costs discouraging people from forming partnerships in the first place? Does "divorce" need a rebranding? Or do those exit costs encourage people to endure the obstacles that inevitably appear in a relationship, despite our naive expectation that a marriage can absorb all stressors? Is it wrong to be held accountable for life's disappointments? It's complex.

I'm searching for a takeaway, a lesson that will endure. Is marriage better than divorce? I think the answer is yes.

Having a spouse or life partner whom you not only care for and want to have sex with, but who's also a good teammate, softens the rough edges, and magnifies the shine of life, is one of life's biggest blessings. I have several friends with impressive careers, supportive friends, and spouses they love. But they aren't happy, because their spouses aren't their partners. Their goals and approaches to life are out of sync. Misalignment on what's important and a lack of appreciation for the other person makes everything so much harder. My friends with less economic success who spend less time with friends but who have real partners to share their struggles and successes with are tangibly happier.

FINALLY . . .

I see marriage through a male lens (can't help that) and present the following toast as advice to the guy on being a good husband and partner.

Don't Keep Score

It's human nature to inflate your own contribution to the relationship and minimize your partner's. Couples who are always taking notes on who's done what for whom waste energy, and ultimately both feel as if they're in the loss column. Decide if the relationship, on the whole, gives you joy and comfort, and if it does (and it better, at this point), then commit to always being on the positive side of the ledger: aim to be generous and do as much for your partner as often as possible. Be willing to wipe the slate clean if and when your partner messes up, as your partner will. Studies show that forgiveness is a key attribute to sustainable, happy relationships. One of the main components of our success as a nation is we give people a second chance. It's no different in relationships—achieving real love and a sense of partnership will likely involve forgiveness that, at the time, feels unfair and even embarrassing.

As we get older, we get more reward from giving. Keeping score creates a dynamic where you never give in to the real joy in life: doing something for someone because you love them, and choosing their happiness over everything else, full stop. Caregivers are the most important contributors to the species and, despite the stress and strain often involved, have lower mortality rates than non-caregivers. Marriage is a promise to give care, every day.

Don't Ever Let Your Wife Be Cold or Hungry

I mean . . . ever. In retrospect, most of the really awful fights I've had with partners have been because we managed to skip lunch. Invest in dual-zone climate control cars, and when you sit down at a restaurant, before you do anything, ensure you are not dining with Satan—a draft of cold air. Never leave the house without energy bars and one of those oversized cashmere scarves that could double as a blanket. You're welcome.

Express Affection and Desire as Often as Possible

Affection, touch, and sex reinforce that your relationship is singular. That this person, when all else is stripped away, is who you want. We are animals, and affection and sex are where you can be most who you really are. People who don't feel desired are more likely to feel insecure and to like themselves less around you, which can metastasize into a variety of relationship cancers. According to Drs. John and Julie Gottman of the Gottman Institute, authors and psychologists who research couples and relationships, the so-called Four Horsemen (contempt, criticism, defensiveness, and stonewalling) are leading predictors of early divorce. Ditto for emotional withdrawal. Note: 85 percent of all stonewallers in heterosexual relationships are men.

Without someone to share your life, professional achievements, and family with, though, you've seen a ghost—it sort of happened, but not really. However, with the right partner, these things feel real, you feel more connected to the species, and all "this" begins to register meaning. Love is what it's all about.

chapter 8

FATHERHOOD

NAUSEA

In 2007, my girlfriend got pregnant, and I witnessed the profoundly disturbing miracle of birth as my son rotated out of her. I felt pretty much none of the things you're supposed to feel: love, gratitude, wonder. I could barely stand. Mostly I felt nausea and panic at the science experiment we were embarking on to keep this thing alive.

However, as it often does, instinct kicked in, and the experiment became less awful, even likable. Unconditional love took over.

With procreation out of the way, the need to protect and provide grew increasingly intense when I became a father. When the financial crisis that year hit, it hit me hard. I went from sort of wealthy to most definitely not. The previous financial crisis had registered the same economic effect, but it had rolled right off me, as I was in my early thirties and knew I could take care of myself. But this was different. I had made a lot of money, but I'd invested most of it in RedEnvelope. I followed the advice of the venture capital community: if you're talented and a baller, you need to go all in. In a three-week period in 2008, the stock went from $7 to Chapter 11. My net worth went from

$10 million to $12 million to negative $2 million, since I was one of those idiots who'd borrowed against their stock to buy even more stock. Then my oldest son had the poor judgment to come marching out of my girlfriend. My first emotion was that I'd failed to live up to my responsibility as a man; i.e., to take care of my child. Not being able to provide for the needs of a kid in Manhattan the way I had envisioned for my son seriously fucked with my sense of why I was here (as in, on earth) and my worth as a man. I was shaping up to fail on a cosmic level, and the flame of hunger burned brighter.

The pressure many men put on themselves to be good providers is irrational. The instinct to protect and nurture your offspring is core to the success of our species. However, believing your kid must have Manhattan private schools and a loft in Tribeca is your ego, not paternal instincts. You can be a good, even great dad on a lot less than I thought I needed to earn. Nonetheless, some of my insecurities I hadn't fully faced arose and I felt deficient as a provider right away.

Whenever I didn't have money as a single, childless person, I could always figure out ways to make it back. There was always enough to eat brunch at cool places or own a luxe TV and speaker system. I never worried. But once my kid came, life felt scarier and more tenuous. This was coupled with the realization it wasn't about me anymore. The fairly selfish person who enjoyed his freedom—maybe a bit too much—was gone. If you plan on being a reasonable dad, the life you were leading and the person you were before kids come dies. It's a mercy killing—don't sweat it. I was used to lots of people around me, and doing what I wanted when I wanted to, and suddenly those were gone.

Also, I hadn't been good at relationships. I worried that if I fucked up this one, it would have an exponentially bigger impact. Specifically, I was now responsible for a kid, and it freaked me out. This is probably natural. I didn't have a role model and knew I wanted to do differently than how my father had raised me. In many ways this fear was motivating and productive—my economic security has grown exponentially since the birth of my oldest. Was this a function of newfound focus or a raging bull market? Yes.

If I wasn't instantly in love, I fell in love over time. At first my only job was to keep the thing alive, and the upside wasn't readily apparent. If you hear angels singing and see bright lights, great. If not, don't worry, it comes.

Note: *New fathers almost always feel unprepared for being dads, and that's normal.*

IN THE BEGINNING

We pretend parenthood is immediately fun. It's not. A dad's job is to show up, do night feedings, change diapers, make sure his wife gets some sleep and keeps her sanity, and do what he can do to make the home feel secure, her loved, and the new baby comforted. Be a ballast—a steadying force, focused, and disciplined about money to avoid that stress infecting the household. Also, just be there.

New dads' testosterone levels drop by a third, beginning during their partners' pregnancies. Their balls shrink, too. An evolutionary logic is at work here—testosterone works great if you're competing for mates, but it's incompatible with caring for and bonding with babies. There's a quietude, a relaxation, in thinking about someone else; it's probably a function of lower T. I enjoyed my weekends as a single guy, but they were stressful, too. How could I optimize them to take advantage of my single, successful, fabulous self? When you're a dad, brunch is exposed as the dumb, made-up thing it is. It's not about what cool people you're hanging with; it's about Johnny's birthday party. Yes, for the first couple of years, being a dad could be frustrating and boring at times, but then it became strangely relaxing to know exactly what I was going to do on the weekends—soccer matches, rewatching *Despicable Me*, picking up after messes. There's a comfort in having the same answer to most of life's questions: whatever is best for the kids. People without kids bask in the same light when they're kind and caring to others.

If you have the flexibility and resources, I would have a second one sooner rather than later. Having two felt three or four times better than one. One is too much pressure and focus—on you and the kid. I was an only child and believe I missed a lot. The negotiation, arguments, balance, positive tension that happens between siblings or even between parents and kids—the joy, stress, noise, and motion that two kids bring to a household—feels like the difference between having a cool accessory and having a family. I'm glad we have two. I wish we'd had another, but I was worried about money and felt we were pushing our luck. It's a challenging world for kids, and I felt we should cash out with two wonderful boys. Looking back, I wish we'd had a daughter, too, but it wasn't in the cards.

There is an arc to happiness. Across every culture, happiness looks like a smile: youth is (mostly) about *Star Wars*, football, and discovering limits with friends and with yourself. And . . . slowly, then suddenly, you get less happy, as kids and careers are stressful. The realization you're not going to be a senator or have a fragrance named after you is a bummer. Generally speaking, people are their least happy

The Arc of Happiness

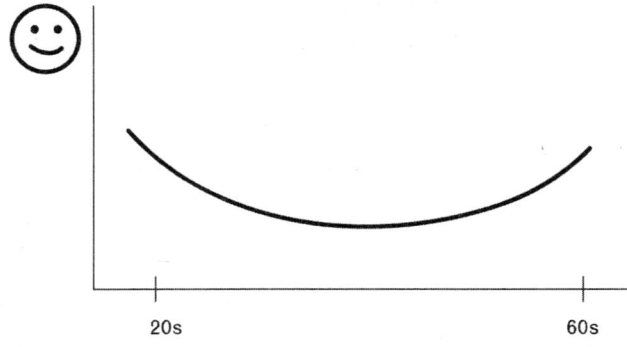

from the ages of twenty-five to forty-five. So, if you feel stressed, unhappy even, recognize that you're tracking. That's part of the journey.

Before kids, for me, there was never enough . . . I was always hungry for more. More money, more fabulous experiences, more relationships, more impressive people, more relevance . . . more. The pursuit always managed to distract me, and I was unable to get the engines of success and fulfillment firing on all cylinders. This stage of my life was characterized by fits of progress, getting close but never achieving anything resembling the potential my opportunities warranted. In one moment that all changed for me when we had a kid, then another. There are moments now with my sons when I think, *This is it, I'm good.*

Having a kid is also the ultimate expression of optimism and commitment to your partner: whether you like it or not, you're committing to stay in each other's lives for eighteen-plus years. Keep in mind, your relationship with your kids' mother will be the reference for how they will likely treat their adult partners. See above: be there. In sum, having kids was the best thing I've done that ruined my life.

> **Note:** *Having kids is the best thing you can do that will ruin your life.*

TAKING AFFECTION BACK

In a 2017 piece published on Medium, Mark Greene, an author and podcaster, argued that affection has been taken away from males—and that's hurting us all. I believe him. As boys, we're trained that affection is either a means of progressing to sex or a sign of homosexuality—which was, when and where I grew up, a bad thing. Because of these associations—unwelcome sexual motives or homoeroticism—our touch is not trusted, so most males are robbed of affection. It's lost from our arsenal of expressions to signal friendship, fondness, or love. As I get older, I've made a conscious effort to take affection back, especially as it relates to my boys. It bonds us, and I'm fairly certain it will add confidence to their lives and years to mine.

One way is kissing. My friend Lee comes from an Italian family. His dad owned furniture stores and looked like Burt Reynolds's younger brother. Lee Sr. had come to San Francisco to visit Lee after he'd moved up to join me at my first firm, Prophet. What I remember most about that day was when Lee Sr. first showed up. He walked into the apartment, and he and Lee Jr. kissed . . . on the lips, as if they were shaking hands. I had never seen two grown men kiss before. Twenty years later my other touchstone for Italian culture, *The Sopranos*, confirmed this is common practice. I remember, after the initial shock, thinking it was nice.

I kiss my boys a lot, though more when they were younger. The act itself is nice, but the real reward is the respect my boys have for the moment. They can be watching TV, fighting, complaining (they complain a shit-ton), but when I signal the kiss (I lean in and pucker), they stop everything, angle their chin upward, and kiss me on the lips . . . and then go back to what they were doing. It's as if they know this has meaning—the other stuff can wait a few seconds.

Another way I showed affection when they were little is holding hands. And, funny enough, I never enjoyed holding hands until I had kids. The things we do for our kids—the soccer practices, the worry, the carpools, the bad movies, setting up remote controls, working to give them a better life than ours: in isolation, each of these things is okay—tolerable—but nothing anybody who doesn't have kids would ever do. (Have you seen *The Emoji Movie*?) Together, though, they give you the sense you're serving a larger purpose.

Few things encapsulate this reward and distill it into a single action more than holding your child's hand. Every kid's hand fits perfectly into their parent's. It's one of those moments when you feel that if you were to drop dead, it would be bad but far less tragic than if you had not marked the universe with purpose and success. You're a parent, and your kid is holding your hand.

At some point, my oldest began holding my hand less—the stirrings of his independence. At least he didn't freak out and scream "Stop it!" like the fourteen-year-old girl I once overheard on the soccer field whose mom had committed the crime against humanity of grabbing her teenage daughter's hand. My guess is, later the daughter felt bad.

But my then seven-year-old son still instinctively grabbed my hand whenever we went outside, and it was magical. At home, he was a barbarian, terrorizing us all. But out in the wild he was a bit intimidated and wanted the security of touch from someone he knew would protect him. He dove for his mom's hand first. I was runner-up ... and that was okay.

I started registering the individuality of my parents when I was his age. Parents are like consumer brands in that, as kids, we remember only two or three key things about them, missing the nuance you only appreciate as you get older and realize people are complicated. My mom was smart, loved me, and was no-nonsense. My dad was intense and quiet around us as a family, but uber-charming and outgoing around strangers.

Hard to speculate what your kids will remember about you when they're older. I've inherited some of the anger and intensity of my father, which makes our home less light than it could be. But I'm committed to ensuring that some of my kids' associations with me are "always kissing us, always extending his hand."

> **Note:** *Model physical affection as often as possible with your kids. It's magical.*

JUST ENGAGE

The best periods of my life have been defined by engagement, and my worst moments by lack of it. As a dad, you need to find moments of engagement with your boys, my book agent Jim Levine suggested once. This stuck with me. As I have no real manly skills (fishing, hunting, building fences) to bond with my kids over, I opt for the cheap route and establish intimacy with my sons by breaking rules. I picked this up from my dad. At nine, my youngest son began easing into mild mischief with his dad, but his twelve-year-old brother would have none of it. The youngest and I drank Coke when their mom was out. I had a stash. The oldest lectured us on how much sugar—which apparently causes inflammation—is in the Atlanta champagne.

I had some success getting my oldest to watch R-rated movies with me, but he demanded we fast-forward through the sex scenes. Gratuitous violence was okay, which is something. Note: *Deadpool* is the only R-rated movie we've watched, but still . . . R-rated.

I thought we were on the verge of a breakthrough last year when, after hibachi, the valet brought our car. As my youngest got in the back, he asked why there was a child seat. I realized, almost immediately . . . it wasn't our car.

"It's not our car! But it is now!" I barked, leaning forward. I threw it into drive. "Where do you want to go?!"

My youngest, the crazy one, seemed on board for about two, maybe three seconds. Enough time to say, "Orlando!" But as younger brothers do, he checked his emotions and poked his head through the middle of the front seats to scope out his brother's reaction. On his brother's face was uncontaminated terror.

"No, Dad, you're going to get us in trouble!" So, fun Dad had become scary Dad . . . not a great feeling. I got about fifty feet before our car-boosting crew had a change of heart, and we returned the car to the valet. Based on my son's reaction, I thought the valet might be angry. When I got out of the car I attempted to say it was "a wee mishap" in a Scottish accent. Only my Scotch sounds like a dead language twins speak to each other, or what I might sound like mid-stroke.

I don't buy that there's an afterlife, so I believe my only shot is to establish a set of relationships that are singular. Isn't that what we all want? To have people you love remember you as someone who, for them, there was no other. Someone they think of often—your image, your smell, your mannerisms, your oddities. Singular. I hope they'll understand me. But more than understanding, I want them to miss me, terribly.

As a man I've tended to be more focused on solutions, and on fixing, rather than listening. Other people's feelings, especially women's feelings, have often been overwhelming for me. Did not want them to feel any negative emotion, especially on my account. Always managing, versus investing and partnering. To get to the other end takes skill—tools I wasn't taught as a young man and that I'm trying to learn now and am committed to learning the rest of my life.

On my podcast, I once interviewed the philosopher and neuroscientist Sam Harris. I asked him for one piece of advice on how to be a better man. He offered that rather than trying to parent, cajole, discipline, or guide your children, your real purpose is just . . . to love them. My youngest son had a hard time during Covid. I spent less time correcting, explaining, arguing, and more just loving . . . sitting in his room when he was doing homework, engaging in conversation, and watching *The Simpsons* together. We got up to season 5; as of this writing, there are 36.

> **Note:** *Find as many moments of engagement with your kids as you can. Your real purpose is just to love them.*

A NICE PLACE TO VISIT

In episode 28 of *The Twilight Zone*, "A Nice Place to Visit," a criminal finds himself in heaven, where he can never lose. So he gets bored—when winning means nothing, he realizes he's actually in hell. Winning may boost dopamine, but only when losing is a constant.

As my boys got older, I began losing a lot. I commute for work and increasingly, when I came home, my kids didn't even look up from the dinner table. My oldest often queried Alexa rather than his dad. Most overtures, questions, comments, observations, went to Mom.

But there still were the intermittent rewards that got me hooked on the whole kids' thing. Three nice hits of dopamine from when my boys were six and nine that have stayed with me:

- We were in London and had the boys in soccer camp (when in Rome). Walking through Hyde Park, I was charged with fetching my youngest when he spotted me and shouted to the other six-year-olds on the field, "There's my dad, look how big he is!" Pretty sure he meant it in a good way. He then ran over to me and, uncharacteristically, jumped into my extended arms.
- We were watching *Monster Jam* when my nine-year-old began stroking my head. He likes the way it feels after I've shaved it (go figure). Unsolicited affection from your children is about as close to the definition of authentic there is—no motive, no planning, no agenda . . . just raw, instinctive affection.
- I was home after traveling and had put my sons to bed. My oldest put in his Invisalign, lay down next to me, and drifted off in my arms. I couldn't help but stare at this thing that sort of looked, smelled, and felt like me, but so much newer and better. Suddenly he stirred and began to smile. He opened his eyes and told me he and his buddies did an improv play at school and it was "hilarious." He drifted back to sleep. He was warm, safe, loved, and next to a dad who wondered if he (like his

dad) was unremarkable but might still (like his dad) have remarkable opportunities.

PURPOSE-DRIVEN

I've been thinking a lot over the last ten years, trying to figure out my purpose. For so long, my only purpose was to be rich and awesome and go to parties where I would be surrounded by rich, awesome people. And I wanted more. As everyone knows, more is an addiction that feeds on itself. You don't appreciate what you have, since once you scale one peak, you focus on climbing the next.

Having kids changed that for me. Here's an example. Recently, I was in London, sitting on the couch, watching the Premier League. Chelsea was playing someone else. The dogs rolled in and joined me on the couch. Then both my boys rolled in, too. Instinctively, they threw their legs over mine. These boys were no longer elves, either. My oldest is now sixteen, and six feet, all arms and legs, and his little brother is thirteen. For a moment, what's happening on TV is totally irrelevant. *This is it*, I think. *This is all that matters.*

You might think the *more* reflex would get triggered. But it doesn't. I can't imagine having more children. Or more dogs. Or more legs. This is it. For the first time, and this happens regularly with me these days, I feel I've been handed permission to leave this world feeling like a success. All my ridiculous desires and wants and fantasies feel sated and/or sutured. It's like religion. Being with my family is like the world's smallest possible congregation. So how do I add surplus value? And how do I figure out a way to raise confident, decent young men? Being in those moments with them when we're relaxed and affectionate and unself-conscious feels godly.

I'm working on being a parent who communicates principles of kindness, empathy, and perseverance instead of assuming they'll organically show up in my boys because they wear smart uniforms to school and have good teachers. I recently had dinner with the CEO of a Fortune 500 firm, and we spent most of our time talking about our kids. His experience and advice was that kids are listening. Even if it's a decade later, and there's just an echo of your counsel, they are listening. This resonated, but I realized you need to be saying something for them to be listening. So I'm coaching and reminding . . . a lot. After soccer, I tell my oldest I noticed him using his left foot well, and that it's good in life to use all the resources you have available. That if he burns up too much energy early in the game, he won't push through the harder second half. Steadiness, resilience, using your energy well—I hope these are life lessons.

THE LAG

These days, my oldest responds to most of my questions with monosyllabic answers. I continue to ask, as occasionally I get a full sentence back. Sometimes he'll even initiate a conversation, and I become flustered with excitement, as if an alien is reaching out to talk to me. Even though they appear indifferent, we tell our boys when they're messing up because they're listening. There's just a lag to them hearing what you're saying. Every fourth game, I play Sushi Go! with them, as I trust when they're older they'll recognize this card game is, for adults, so awful as to be just short of an enhanced interrogation technique.

Our youngest once came into our bed two to three times a week. During the day he took great care to fight me . . . on everything. I mean everything. However, reengaging, at night he stumbled to our room and, similar to a peace offering, straddled me as if hugging a tree. I would wait a few minutes, then roll counterclockwise and spill him into the center of the bed and put my hand on his back, so he knew he was part of a pack. He drifted off. He wasn't just sleeping, but dreaming, processing, learning, and growing—1.5 millimeters each night. He was asleep. It's just that this process had a similar effect on his dad as a cold plunge pool, and I was now very much awake. The cold plunge set in motion the process of getting up, peeing, walking around the house, checking on his brother, maybe peeing again, and not sleeping. I may not have gotten the sleep back, but I could still recapture the hours, as I'll be around longer. I'm engaged.

The only profound thing I've ever done is to partner with and love someone, and together bring into the world, and love, two boys. The work, the fake relevance, the money, is all a means to the ends. My ends used to wear Iron Man and Darth Vader pajamas. Still, I find time to turn inward, shut them out, and focus on what's not right with my life (approximately 0.1 percent). I'm anxious and digress into feeling sorry for myself—can't stand this tendency.

A few weeks ago, my youngest fell ill. We knew something was wrong, as he became . . . nice. Most days, my youngest spends his time assessing weaknesses and vulnerabilities in the household. It's as if strangers have invaded—his mom, dad, and brother. He is bold and deeply committed to an ideology we don't understand. He strikes when we least expect it. He's our insurgent.

But that day, he was nice, weak, kind, and telling us he loved us. Then he said something nice to his brother. That was it: something was seriously wrong. His fever was skyrocketing, and we took him to the emergency room. They ran tests, told us he had the flu, and sent us home. That night around one a.m. we heard what sounded like an old lady screaming over and over: "SO? SO? SO?" His mom and I ran up to his room. He was sitting up, drenched in sweat, pleading for answers from someone we couldn't see. I sat on the bed in front of him and tried to comfort him:

"It's all right, Nolan, we're here. It's all right."

He grabbed my hands, clenching them like a Nintendo controller, and then looked directly into my eyes but right through me.

"I'm sorry," he said. And again, only louder and more distressed: "I'm sorry!"

Now yelling and incredibly distraught: "I'm sorry, Mom, I'M SORRY!"

We couldn't snap him out of this, and it felt as if we were in a cheap remake of *Poltergeist* or *The Amityville Horror*. But this was definitely not funny. It was frightening.

At that moment, all my other concerns were just narcissism. You just want your kid to be better. Nothing else matters. Nothing else has purchase in your soul. The fires of a need for relevance, worrying about things I couldn't control, or blaming others for my own deficiencies were, for now, arrested. As long as the people I love and who love me are healthy, everything else is just noise.

I lost my self-absorption for a moment and thought about the millions, maybe billions, of people in a constant state of despair over the well-being of their children. Facing, every day, things they can't control, that aren't their fault or their doing, that threaten their kids' well-being. Except it feels like it's your fault. Our only real job here is to ensure our kids survive and prosper. Any threat to this survival and hopeful prosperity is the ultimate failure. It cuts to tissue and emotions you didn't know existed.

We walked our youngest downstairs in an attempt to break him from his night terror. He calmed and fell asleep. We debated for an hour if we should go back to the emergency room but decided to let him sleep in our bed, taking his temperature every half hour. The next day we watched him like a hawk. He still wasn't well, but he wasn't levitating, spinning his head, or speaking in tongues.

The following morning his brother couldn't find the remote. After searching for twenty minutes and giving up, our recently possessed son reached into his underwear, pulled out two AA Duracell batteries, and chucked them at his brother's face. He then announced he wouldn't brush his teeth that day. He wouldn't be eating again, ever, as we didn't cook broccoli right. A wave of relief. He was better. The insurgent was back.

SELF STUPID

My iPhone keeps serving pictures of my boys from years ago. It is very rewarding and, at the same time, heartbreaking. I feel a rush of happiness, and then longing sets in. I will never have back the five-year-old who let me grow his curls out. Gone is the eight-year-old who'd sleep naked unless you found pajamas with Jedi Master Yoda on them. If you don't find the preceding two sentences nauseating, it means one thing: you have kids.

I'm with my boys in New York. The oldest is . . . gone. He's figured out that I'm not that cool and seems angry I let the charade go on this long. His favorite thing is, when out with his dad, to ask if he can walk home alone and leave several minutes before me. I know he'll come back, and friends told me to expect it, but I am still shocked how fast the eye roll arrived.

His younger brother, that's a different story. We went to the Edge, an observation deck in Hudson Yards where, for $38 each, you and a couple thousand tourists get to look at the city from one hundred floors up. This, for me, is the seventh ring of hell. However (pro tip for dads), I recognize that moments of engagement with my sons are a function of getting into what they are interested in.

He spots the advertised "Thrilling Glass Floor," which we lie down on and take selfies. He then pops up as he has great news: "Dad . . . there's a bar! Should we get Cokes?" I nod, and he sprints, I mean sprints, to the bar, stops, runs back, grabs money from his dad, and sprints back to the bar. Sitting, drinking Atlanta champagne on stone benches, gazing at the city from the tallest human-made outdoor viewing platform in the Western Hemisphere, he looks at me and says, "Isn't this amazing?" This is the closest I will get to heaven.

Later that night, the boys are asleep, I have had a Zacapa and Coke and am feeling emotional. I text some people who mean a lot to me and tell them about my experience that day and how I feel about my sons and fatherhood and what I've gotten right and wrong. They respond, and we're closer. The next morning, with some distance from the moment with my son, I am a bit embarrassed about my texts. I'm glad to share with friends but worry about burdening them with my emotions. A work in progress.

THE MORE-NESS OF LESS

Scarcity taps into our competitive instinct as people strive to meet the criteria being used to determine who gets what. What do Bang & Olufsen speakers, Birkin bags, and your girlfriend moving to Singapore have in common? They're better, or at least the perception is they are better. I find the more speaking gigs I turn down, the more requests I get. The top twenty universities could expand their supply—seats for incoming freshmen—50 percent within the decade. But they won't, as the prestige that stems from scarcity is the ointment for irrelevance that most academics thirst for.

One of the benefits of having kids at a later age is you have a greater understanding of scarcity. Not just of time but of your kids . . . and who they are. One of the things I dislike (most) about myself is too often I feel sorry for myself. I think about this a lot, so I can put an end to this bullshit. Two situations create my one-man pity party:

1. When I'm at an airport and the clusterfuck that's our air transportation system turns my sojourn home into the Bataan Death March—delays, canceled flights, missed flights, etc.

2. When I've been on the road for a couple weeks, and I come home, peek my head into our boys' room, where they are fast asleep, and register that they have grown since the last time I saw them. Really. Bums. Me. Out.

I begin reevaluating my life and start planning the reconfiguration. However, by morning the sobriety of my need for relevance and economic security has downgraded the reconfiguration to driving the kids to school that day.

I hope, however, I'm more "in the moment" by understanding the scarcity of time with my boys.

Your friends, by now, are largely static as people. They will have more expression (lines) in their faces, but you'll generally get the same Bob and Jen next summer as this one. Not true with kids. A few years ago, my oldest was small for his grade, and very attached to his parents... in our bed every morning. A year later, he was four inches taller and prone to rolling his eyes... and didn't come into our room much anymore. Meanwhile, his younger brother didn't coordinate his clothes and often left the house dressed like an angry clown: lots and lots of colors. He had a big mane of curls. I am fascinated by my boys' manes. It's shocking to me we are in the same species, much less father and sons. Now, though, my youngest is suddenly very aware of his outfits, posing in front of the mirror and asking me to comb his hair straight, like his brother's.

The kid you have this summer is leaving... forever. The skinny boy with the lion's mane who tiptoed into our room and, on first evidence of me stirring, would say, "Dad, let's make a plan for the day," is gone. It's incredibly sad. A relative of his will be back next summer, but different. The compensation is that there will be new attributes you find hilarious and endearing. But still, sad.

I put, mentally, a big sign above my boys' heads: LIMITED EDITION, YOUR ELEVEN-YEAR-OLD SON, ONE SUMMER ONLY.

I remember when my oldest son, Alec, left for camp for the first time. I had a strange sensation in my feet, hollow yet tingly, and I was not as much sad as numb, feeling nothing. This is how I experience mild depression. Not sure if the catalyst was my concern for him to be in a new environment—he's social but a bit awkward—or that, more likely, this was a marker of time. My mind quickly jumped to *I'm going to die soon.*

Time and progress have been for me like the Big Wheel that populates the fronts of casinos: my mom's hand on it, and that of the University of California, got the wheel moving. Morgan Stanley, grad school, luck, hard work, America, the internet era, and cheap capital really got the wheel spinning. But now that I've finally arrived where I was trying to get—meaningful relationships, relevance, economic security—the wheel won't slow. Time is, as it does, becoming smaller relative to an increasingly broad horizon—the amount of time I've been here—and years are beginning to feel like months.

An atheist, I've convinced myself that I experience time as more finite than most, since I'm convinced the last time I look my loved ones in the eyes I will know our relationship is over—we won't be reunited.

This. Is. It.

Note: I acknowledge I can be as obnoxious about my atheism as any zealot, and that the notion of an afterlife isn't any more ridiculous than my view that in the beginning there was nothing, then a big explosion. But that's a subject for another time.

I have only a handful of more holidays with my boys, and twenty or thirty more with everyone else. Again, the hollow-feet feeling. So, how to slow time's relentless march? Humans are good at guessing the time, always have a decent sense of what time it is, but don't perceive it well—our brain registers time at different speeds. David Eagleman, neuroscientist and foremost researcher on time perception, believes time is a construction of the brain, and our minds filter the info before presenting it to us. When we experience fear, pleasure, or novelty, our senses become heightened. Our brain stands at attention and records more information, slowing time.

For the last few years I've been using an app, One Second Everyday, that lets you capture (you guessed it) one second of video each day. I miss half the days, so forty years from now I'll have around two hours of video. I plan to be at home, surrounded by loved ones, and then am going to experiment with hallucinogens and live my life over, in two-hour increments, several times.

DOING WHAT DAD DOES

Growing up, I was fascinated by all things Dad. I played golf and soccer as a child—neither of which I had much natural interest in, but my dad did. I wanted to be closer to and impress him, and that meant doing what he was interested in. I would tag along to the golf course just to be around him. I didn't have innate soccer talent, but I became a decent golfer. About twenty years ago, my dad got too old to play golf, and I've maybe played three rounds since.

I assumed, reasonably, that my two boys would be as fascinated with me as I was with my dad. More even, since I'm around, available, and supportive. Once I had a vision of the three of us sitting around, discussing CrossFit or watching World War II documentaries while arguing the finer points of antitrust legislation. If my boys weren't into it, they would at least pretend. But, frankly, they're incredibly unimpressed with me and with any of the things I'm interested in.

If I'm being honest, I'm disappointed by their response. I find it heartbreaking, actually. I tell myself I'm such a good dad. I make such an effort with them. Honestly, I'm much more impressive personally and professionally than my dad was. Growing up, I always felt I gave more love to my dad than he gave me. I did my best to impress him. I tried really hard to be a good son, always made a huge effort. Basically, I gave more than I got. My dad wasn't a bad person, but his neglect and lack of responsiveness had me scrambling to fill in the gaps. A tailspin ensued, and I became less engaged at school, felt it incumbent to be the man of the house for my mom, got stressed out about money way too young, and generally felt confused and unsure of my worth—except in the eyes of my mom, who anchored and loved me deeply.

My boys aren't nearly as impressed by me, nor are they as desirous for my approval. The idea of them going somewhere with me for four hours just to hang out? It's not going to happen. They have too much else going on.

At first, I felt like a failure because I didn't have a buddy-buddy relationship with my kids. So I reframed it. Maybe I'm rationalizing this—but it's because they know I'm there. Present. Engaged. Their taking me somewhat for granted is a compliment. It means I've done my job. I'm supposed to end up in the minus column. That's what being a good dad means. Countering my disappointment that they aren't more impressed with me, or proud of me, or hungry for my approval, is the fact they know they have it. They know I'm always there for them, thinking, worrying about them. You might say they haunt me. Hands down, they're my priority.

Pro tip for dads: your kids don't inherit your interests; it's your job to foster and adopt theirs. If you don't get interested in what your kids are into, you won't have much overlap. Truth is, I never cared much for soccer or sports in general. But my sons love it, so I love it, and now we go to Premier League football games in different cities all the time. Only now that we live in London, we call it football. I played twice one weekend in the backyard with my oldest, and a week later I was with both sons at the Emirates Stadium watching Arsenal play Wolves.

I don't watch the game so much as I register moments that inspire my boys. I observe their reactions. I hope I'm alive when they have kids, so we can share, and discuss, the intensity and range of emotions you have for your children. Soccer provides some of those moments. They call it "the Beautiful Game." Maybe. What's clear is that soccer offers us something increasingly scarce: an in-person experience where men are encouraged to express their emotions and bond with one another. While other people and organizations pay billions to feel younger, I'm grateful that I feel closer to my sons.

> **Note:** *Creating surplus value and ending up in the minus column is what being a good dad is all about.*

GIVING/TAKING

As children, my sons get more education and resources from their school and town and country than they give back. I tell them their teachers are doing everything they can to damage the muscle between their ears so it grows back stronger. Children don't pay taxes or help fix potholes, but, even minus that tax revenue, the cops and fire department will still bail them out in a pinch. They don't know how good they have it.

Children who grow up in blessed households often get more love than they give. In London, where we live, my boys can board the tube to go to great schools. There are malls where they can play mini golf. People in general are kinder to kids than adults in part because they're fascinated by them. There's no expectation those kids will be nice in return. The government feels the same. It spends a ton of money on children's healthcare, schools, and free lunch. Kids create zero tax revenue and productivity. Recently, my oldest son was thinking about college. We got him a tutor for the ACT. I asked him if he'd scheduled the first meeting (my wife and I had asked him to do this three hundred times). He shook his head. I got mad. Didn't he know how much time and energy we were spending trying to get him into a decent college—and he couldn't set up an hour to get tutored? At some point a boy needs to figure this out—needs to flip things around and start adding more value than he's taking.

Understanding this was a huge reveal for increasing my own happiness and satisfaction. I used to be transactional. The people who worked for me weren't much more than instruments of economic utility. The same went for my romantic relationships and business partnerships. If the relationship was asymmetrical, I'd get frustrated—I was, I thought, then on the losing side of justice. I did this a lot with my dad, who was never very involved in my life. Ergo, went my thinking, I won't be involved in his. We were even.

That's infantile—and I've moved on. Why would I perpetuate an unhealthy early relationship with my dad in all the other relationships in my life? Especially a relationship that often made me feel like crap. Here's the approach I took once I understood that: What kind of person, citizen, neighbor, spouse, son, father, teacher, and son do

I want to be? *Better* is the answer. If you keep score all the time, invariably moments will arise where you add more value than your colleagues and friends do. If you go around feeling unhappy, pissed off, and vengeful, this isn't healthy. Worse, it prevents you from becoming a man.

Some boys never make the transition to creating surplus value. Concierge, bulldozer, and helicopter parents contribute to more self-indulgent young men than almost any other factor. The eighth-winningest kid lines up to receive a trophy, the phony feel-good school ecosystem with its lack of emphasis on fitness—that version of masculinity is actively bad for young men. It tells them nothing is their fault and they're responsible for their successes but not their failures, that they can sit passively by and still be winning. They get to marinate in negative surplus value their whole lives while believing they're still being good citizens. Bullshit. Occasionally you have to try really hard, and occasionally, despite your best efforts, you'll lose. When that happens, you need to be a man about it—get up, shake it off, and either persevere or congratulate your opponent. The transition from boyhood to manhood and fatherhood means recognizing that it's your job to add more value than you take, across every dimension.

This understanding transformed my relationship to and with my dad and the world. I jettisoned the scorecard. I became, or at least tried to become, a generous, loving man. It unlocked other things, too. For example, I've decided it's okay to overpay people. I like to joke that out of all the employees in my companies over the past two decades, there are a handful of people who are two or three bad decisions away from living in their car. They're not bad at what they do, or drug addicts, or clinically insane, but their work is no more than acceptable or competent. I could find someone else to do their jobs for $12 an hour, not $80,000 plus benefits.

But I decided it's okay to have a few of those people around. Surplus benefit—trying to be a better friend, employer, partner, dad, than your friends, employees, partners, kids, are to you. What kind of husband do I want to be? I want to be a generous, supportive husband who's strong and always there for my partner and makes her feel strong, supported, and loved. With my dad, I decided I wanted to be a generous, loving son regardless of how good or not good he was to me. It made me enjoy our relationship a lot more.

Today, I like spending time with my dad. We share a few qualities, anger being one, self-absorption another, selfishness, money fears, the list goes on. Yes, a lot of negatives here, but the reality is I make my living communicating. Some of that is hard work, the other half is the DNA passed down by my dad. Speaking is the family business. You have to give your parents credit for the DNA whether you want to or not. I'm lucky. That DNA has made me wealthy. It's given my family and me an extraordinary life. Yes, much had to do with my environment, my blessings and privilege, the University of California, my own perseverance. Whatever I ended up with by accident is no reason not to be grateful for and appreciative of it. And to, yes, my dad.

Also, sometimes you'll be cut off in traffic. No rule exists that says a right will be wronged if you don't press down on the horn and holler profanities. Being a man means taking the occasional body blow. It doesn't mean letting other people walk over you, or whack you, but it doesn't have to escalate. Ignore a potential skirmish and it won't become one.

That gives me solace from knowing I give more than I get as a dad. I'd like to think fatherhood is made up of a bunch of nice, tender, fun, rewarding moments. But it's mostly your seventeen-year-old acting like a jerk and you taking it, then defending his mom when he's being even worse to her, if possible, than he is to you.

Being a good dad means asking: Do you feel you're not getting as much back as you give—that you spend more time thinking about your kids than you imagine they think about you? Do you love your kids impossibly much, probably more than they love you? Do you think about them constantly, including what they had for lunch, whether the pillows they sleep on are the correct hypoallergenic mix, or if you filled out the right school forms? If so, you've done your job. That's what being a dad is. You've inched over into the surplus column. It may feel like a loss, but it's not, because everyone wins.

> **Note:** *Don't keep score in your relationships. Instead, be the father, son, and partner you aspire to be.*

DAD LOVES HIS WORK

Home versus work is a core tension of being a provider. Every dad realizes that providing for the people who mean the most to him means disappointing them sometimes. I travel a shit-ton for work. My wife will get angry because my travel schedule means I won't be there to have brunch with her parents on Sunday, or my client meeting in Atlanta conflicts with a school event. I tell her no one is willing to give me a ton of money to stay home and gaze longingly into her eyes. My job is to go out and slay impalas.

The word "breadwinner" goes back to the 1600s, where it referred to any marketable tool, skill, or talent necessary to earn a living. Breadwinning was normalized in the Industrial Revolution, when, for the first time in U.S. history, dads left home to toil en masse in factories. Today, women are the primary breadwinners in 41 percent of U.S. households and the percentage of women who outearn their husbands has tripled in the past fifty years. Among married-couple families with children, 67 percent are ones where both parents work. Both partners working is an increasing reality in American life. This can cause marriages to stumble, especially when fathers refuse to own what they've said they'll do—take the kids to school or the doctor, stock up on house supplies, cook dinner—and see it more as a favor to their partners or wives for which they deserve slavish praise. A smart solution is making unseen labor visible versus implicit/inevitable;

e.g., Mom does the household acquisitioning, Dad cooks dinner three times a week and drives the youngest to daycare. Not a set of favors, in other words, but an outline of expected responsibilities that aims to share the amount of work, house, and kid tasks between both partners equitably.

Being a male provider means making hard decisions on behalf of your family. Experience tells me that instinctively my wife would prefer having me around the house more (she also works but doesn't have to travel nearly as much). But I also need and want to earn a living.

The most stressful periods in my life have been when I'm traveling, speaking, making money, and watching my wealth grow. The times I'm at home, going to the gym, and meeting friends in coffee shops usually coincide with periods when my wealth is declining.

You can have it all, just not all at once. As a man and dad, part of your job is evaluating and managing this trade-off. Sometimes it means leaning into being a provider and coping with feelings of tension and sacrifice. A current narrative is that you'll never regret spending time with your partner and your kids. I agree. But if you really want to stress your wife and kids out, try being broke.

> **Note:** *Work versus family, and who does what, is something every couple faces and needs to figure out together.*

PLEASE DON'T GET USED TO THIS

My mom never made more than $800 a month. Not having money was always a strain. Things have changed. My sons are growing up in ways that were unthinkable to me at their age.

At twelve or thirteen, I used to fly to go visit my dad and Linda in Ohio. My badge ID'd me as an unaccompanied minor. More than four decades later, my wife, two boys, and I were going back and forth from Miami to London—an almost ten-hour flight one way. My wife and I have worked hard to achieve economic security, and we want to fly business class. It's the difference between an uncomfortable flight (business) versus a horrific one (economy). Asking anyone to sit upright for half a day in a pressurized tube is unhealthy, abusive, and gross. In business class, you at least get to stretch out on a flat seat, maybe get some work done. But I don't want my sons to get used to it. They're physically smaller, too, so it matters less. I decided my wife and I should be in business, with the boys in economy.

But the rules have changed. Minors can't sit by themselves unless an adult is present. I ended up buying four business-class seats. As such, we boarded the plane before the other passengers and settled in. My youngest son, having discovered the joys of a reclining seat, was fiddling with the controls as an elderly woman with a walker made her way slowly into economy class. I watched this—my son tearing the plastic off his complimentary Bose headphones while an eighty-five-year-old woman navigated stop-start crowds and a treacherous aisle. It felt sickening and wrong.

Early on, I wanted to take care of my mom. I wanted a broader selection of mates than I probably deserved. I saw money as the path to getting these and more. I worry my boys won't ever have to connect the same dots—that they can work their asses off for the rest of their lives and never come close to living the lives they have now. Because I wouldn't have what I have today if I'd had what they have growing up. This is a privilege problem, but it's a problem.

The only solution: we do our best. As parents, our job is not to traumatize our kids and to be there for them. My wife and I got our boys playing competitive sports early on, for example, in the hope it would teach them lessons about fitness and perseverance. It did. They're both really good kids. But I grapple with how their early lives will shape or possibly deform their future ambition.

One compensation is that, despite the traveling I do, I'm also around. My boys see how much both my wife and I work. No matter where we are, even on vacation, they see I'm on the phone, preparing a podcast, doing research, writing. I like to believe they're taking it all in, that even if they're not connecting the dots I did at their age, new ones are being forged.

GARBAGE TIME

As a man, being a procreator doesn't mean having sex and getting as many women pregnant as possible. It means signing up to raise loving, secure, productive citizens you like being around and spending time with. This usually implies signing up for the company of a partner, too. Kids are deranged, and two adults are better than one.

There's an assumption among divorced men that their scarcity creates "quality time" whenever they see their kids. That's bullshit. Quality time is a concept made up by a bunch of frazzled men who weren't spending enough time with their kids and decided "quality time" compensated for their invisibility. It doesn't.

The author Ryan Holiday came up with a great phrase—garbage time—to describe those random, unplanned times that allow for moments of intimacy between parents and kids. Driving them to school in the morning, running them to soccer practice, cooking dinner together—that's garbage time. It matters . . . a lot. En route to school, out of nowhere your son pipes up that he has a crush on someone. It's the first time you've heard about it. Garbage time happens only when you're around. The rest of the time you're a dork and uncool. But your kids will remember you were there, how your omnipresence made it possible for them to tell you stuff.

That's why being a procreator means you've also signed up for a shit-ton of garbage time. That means you have to figure out how to be around. It's harder if you're a divorced man, as moms are granted custody of the children 80 percent of the time. (Dads, I might add, seldom request full custody, for a variety of reasons). I have a good friend who's a divorced dad. He has two daughters, fourteen and seventeen, whom he loves. But at that age, they're devoted to their friends and to a household infrastructure designed and lubricated by their mom. When their dad shows up on the weekend, it feels like an excise tax. Suddenly, they have to go off and do things with him when they would rather be with their friends. If Dad were around all the time, it wouldn't matter. They could tell jokes over breakfast, go outside and rake some leaves, watch Netflix. My friend knows his girls aren't into him, and it's devastating.

No one was harder on his dad than me until one day I realized that, for all his faults and all my complaints, he was a far better dad to me than his dad had been to him. Ultimately your role as a procreator is to be a better dad to your kids than your dad was to you. This may sound basic, but it's the essence of social evolution.

> *Garbage time—taking drives, hanging out, watching a movie—is what your kids will remember.*

SPEAKING OF DADS...

My dad always made good money. Maybe because he had to—he was married and divorced four times. The first was a woman who followed him from Scotland to Canada. But he started fooling around on her. One day he came home to find her sitting on their couch, impeccably dressed, soaked in vomit. A suicide note hung from a piece of string around her neck. He called EMS, and they took her to the emergency room. He just left her there. She recovered. He never saw her again.

Wife number two was my mom.

Wife number three was a lovely woman named Linda, to whom I'm still fairly close. Linda was the first person to spoil me. She'd been told she couldn't have kids of her own. So when I showed up in my department store corduroys, missing my two front teeth, she was in love. Through Linda, my dad had Asheley, my younger sister and my good friend. Eventually my dad got restless and moved on.

Wife number four was a woman my dad met on a cruise ship. He got a free ticket in exchange for being willing to dance with a dozen women per night. He was a low-end gigolo, basically. My dad was always charming, and older, single women love to sail the seas. His skill, you may have deduced, has always been leaving. When the going got rough, you never saw him again. He went from Glasgow to Toronto, then San Diego. But he needed to find a woman. After Linda, he found a nice woman from Arizona on a cruise who owned trailer parks and proved to be his economic savior. She developed a fairly severe case of Parkinson's after they were twenty-five years married, and he left her. He was eighty-seven. She died two years later. There's no getting around the fact that my dad has shown questionable character and judgment at times. Knowing the end is near, Asheley and I recently put our heads together and tried to envisage a memorial service. "What would be the point?" I said. "He's outlived everyone." Besides us, I couldn't imagine a single person showing up, aside from his caregiver, whom I pay.

At the same time, my dad took risks, he was smart and talented, and in return he's had a pretty great (material) life, certainly better than the lives of his siblings. He had a home near the beach, drove a nice car, flew business class, had fun, danced with widows on oceans, and spread his seed to the four corners of the earth. On a more cosmic level, he will probably die alone in hospice surrounded by angelic nurses and not much else. This was the version of masculinity I grew up with and was determined to do differently, though do take note of his successes and the traits I get from him that contribute to mine.

Two years ago, I took my sons to see the Glasgow Rangers play St. Johnstone in Perth, Scotland. I wanted my soccer-mad sons to see my dad's favorite team in a ten-thousand-seat stadium. I was trying to re-create a memory my dad used to tell me about, when he and his father went to this same game—the Rangers were his team. He'd get emotional talking about that day, one of his few memories of doing something, alone, with his father. When I told my dad about our trip, he didn't remember who the Rangers were. He's in his mid-nineties now, and struggling. As his attention and memories are disappearing, I'm riddled with questions that will likely never be answered. Suddenly, a ton of questions.

CRUSHING IT

We go on vacation sometimes with another family. My older son has a thing for the other dad—he finds him extremely impressive. My friend knows this and likes it—and who wouldn't?—as it's flattering. Sometimes the two of them will go off and do something together. At first, I didn't like this one bit. Frankly, I was jealous. Another spear through the heart. The problem, of course, wasn't that the other dad was unworthy or unimpressive, because he is, but that my son seemed more taken with him than with me.

Then I flipped, grew up, possibly both. Instead of problematic, I began thinking of it as not only nice but important, transitional. At a certain age, kids instinctually pull away from you. The need to separate is stronger than their need to connect and engage. This is easier for them to do if they cool on you first. My boys love and respect me, but for the most part they don't know what I do for a living and could care less. They're at an age where their dad is sort of pitiful and their friends aren't. Friends wash in, you wash out. This will make saying goodbye easier when the time comes.

Most mammals will give their lives defending their offspring.

What makes us human is not just opposable thumbs but also our ability to cooperate. Cooperation draws on what makes us uniquely human, like speech, culture, and long childhoods. One of the most noble forms of cooperation that advances the species is caring for those who aren't biologically yours. I don't enjoy my kids a lot of the time and don't enjoy others' offspring most of the time. It's a miracle people agree to love kids who don't smell, look, or feel like them. Death, disease, and divorce leave a lot of kids in single-parent households, where the odds are markedly worse for them.

The fastest blue-line path to a better world isn't economic growth or a better phone. It's more men becoming irrationally passionate about the well-being of a child who isn't their own, getting involved in the life of a young man. Boys especially have a built-in hormone that causes them to stop listening to their parents, which usually kicks in around the age of fifteen. If you're not their parents, they're much more willing to listen to you. So coaches, uncles, teachers, Dad's best friend, all become important to be around and step up. It's fatherhood by proxy. I probably get fifteen to twenty people a month asking if I'll mentor their sons. I say yes, knowing most other men when asked would say no. They worry they'll be tagged as predators. Thanks to Michael Jackson and the Catholic Church, people are suspicious of an older man taking an interest in a younger man's life. Mentorship has been pathologized. It's now unsafe and creepy.

As a dad, it's striking how easy it is to add value to my own sons' lives. Put on shoes before you go to school. Finish your homework. With friends' children, it's about showing up, being a good listener and role model. (I do this for my kids, too.)

Being a man means acquiring the strength and skills—physical and mental fitness, and economic viability—you need so you can advocate for others. It means taking care of yourself first, followed by your immediate and/or extended family, then moving on to other people and your community. It means being the role model you wish there were more of in the world. If we want better men, we need older men to step up. Getting involved in the life of a boy or young man is the ultimate expression of masculinity and should be welcomed instead of distrusted. In New York, there are three times as many adult applicants to become Big Sisters as there are to become Big Brothers. We need to create a social zeitgeist whereby if a man is doing well, he should feel compelled to cast his eyes down the mountain and assist those who are a quarter of the way up, some maybe out of breath. Mentorship programs are rife in the corporate world—so why not in the real world, too?

The good news is that needy and deserving young men are everywhere. Single mothers especially are looking for men to engage in their sons' lives. It's not unnatural; it's natural. Boys will listen to their dads' friends more than they will their own dads. You don't have to be a baller or some amazing dude—just someone who's trying to lead a good life and can pass on even half of what he knows.

> **Note:** *A successful man needs to get involved in the life of a boy or young man. Kids will often listen to their parents' adult friends more than their parents.*

SHOCKED

One night with friends, we played a game called TableTopics. Players pick a random card and answer a question as sincerely as possible. These aren't lightweight questions; they're closer to deathbed confessions, designed to make you pause or even tear up. *What is your greatest regret?* and *What would you do over if you could?* and *What is the one thing in the future you hope happens?* It's like being in therapy but in card form.

We went around the room. When it was my oldest son's turn, the card he picked asked, *Who do you admire most in the world?* A beauty pageant question, ripe for some bullshit response. My son hesitated. Then he said, "It sounds weird, and like a cliché. It's my dad. My dad is a really great storyteller." He met my eyes briefly, embarrassed, and looked away, and then it was on to the next player.

It was nice, it was moving as hell—but mostly I was shocked. My honest response was *God, I didn't even think you* liked *me*. I feel my boys love me but otherwise I'm a waste of their time. I have to coerce them into hanging out with me, by shuttling them to some kind of fantasy experience you might win on a 1970s game show, a recent one being flying to Barcelona to see FC Barcelona play against Madrid. Frankly, I just couldn't believe what my son had said.

A few months earlier, I'd been asked to speak at his school. When I told him, my son said he wasn't all that comfortable with me doing that; it would embarrass him. Another spear through my heart. The chance to show him what I was good at in front of him and his classmates—what could be more exciting? I begged off, but I was hurt.

My youngest son, Nolan, comes home sometimes and spews his emotions onto his mom. It happens the second he sees her. He can be mean, unreasonable, whiny—awful—but it's because he feels so infinitely comfortable around her. She's his world, his ibuprofen, his Neosporin, his shock absorber, the patch to his busted rowboat. He will summon everything he has at his disposal and lay it on her. Why? Because he knows she'll take it—she and I love him that unconditionally. Last year I flew to Brazil and gave a speech before three thousand people. Toward the end, I had them all shout "Hello, Nolan!" Later, I met the captain of the Brazilian football team. I sent Nolan both videos and FaceTimed him, as I do every night when I'm traveling. "What?" he said, as if I'm a spam call. Distracted by his hair, or some app, it's how he usually answers when he knows it's me.

What the hell do I need to do to impress or engage you? I thought. Nothing is the answer. His mom and I won't put up with rudeness, but anything else our boys can think to hurl at us is fair game. We love them that much—always will. That's surplus value. Parenthood isn't a father-son ad for Gillette Fusion razors or a Hallmark movie with snowflakes falling outside the steamed glass of a bakery. It's a negative game. Giving more love to your kids than they give back to you is what's supposed to happen here. Sure, being a dad is rewarding, sometimes immensely. But you'll never get as much out of it as your kids do. It took me a while to figure this out. When I did, it made sense, and I loved it, and them, more for it.

chapter 9

MAN...NERS

Key to humans' survival is and has been kindness, consideration, and cooperation.

Status-seeking was, too. Thus manners came along, which were how kings, queens, and other nobility distinguished themselves from the masses. During the regime of Louis XIV in the seventeenth century, courtiers traveled to Versailles to curry favor. Many were clods who trampled the royal gardens. The court handed out "tickets" to define where in the gardens courtiers should and shouldn't walk. "Ticket" became "etiquette." This concept spread across Europe and followed the Puritans to New England. In America, manners were seen as a tool of social mobility, good for building reputations and advancing professionally. Not much has changed.

Etiquette books aimed at men historically emphasized honor, leadership, and sacrifice. Young men were encouraged and expected to facilitate conversation, avoid controversy, and serve as champions, lovers, and protectors of women. Manners also underlie the armed services. Clean uniforms, teamwork, and respect for hierarchies and rituals while all manner of crap is being flung at you are qualities that separate soldiers from civilians. The military is also an engine of social mobility.

In 1970s California, etiquette found its way inside an eight-hundred-square-foot-apartment in Westwood.

My mom used to hammer me on manners and hygiene—it was the Brit in her, the mom, or both. At the dinner table, even in a group of people, her lips would purse, reminding me to keep my mouth closed while chewing. She was my own in-house quality assurance inspector. If my nails were dirty, my breath fragrant, my hair unwashed, or if I needed deodorant, she always let me know. I was expected to shower and wash my hair every morning, and she even bought me aftershave. Somehow, she always found money to buy me nice clothes—she wanted me to feel good about myself. She spent more on me than she did on herself.

That left our living space. On Saturdays I could do whatever I wanted, but the first half of every Sunday was always spent sweeping, polishing, and vacuuming. I wasn't allowed to leave or do anything fun unless my bedroom was spotless.

My dad was less of a stickler. For him, manners had more to do with decorum and readiness. He'd joined the Royal Navy at seventeen, and the lessons from his time there stuck.

It brings me little joy to report that my wife and I have failed our boys from a housekeeping perspective. We ask them to do almost nothing except to do well in school and occasionally clean up after the dogs. Chores are important—my sons don't do any. They don't even make their own beds, because they're usually running late in the morning. Both are happy to do stuff if we ask, but . . . we almost never ask. We don't ask much, because by the time the boys get home, they're already so overprogrammed and overscheduled—language tutor, soccer practice . . .

What we do insist on are basic good manners. "This is what a man does," I tell them before coming out with one axiom or another.

At first, they greeted this with annoyed bemusement. But say something enough times and the man . . . ner muscle, responding to sheer reps, breaks down and takes on definition. That's the goal at least.

Good man . . . ners have nothing to do with shooting birds out of the sky or going to Ascot. Good manners are manhood in action. They communicate respect. They show that you have a core, a code, show that you're disciplined and organized, and that you anticipate and consider others before yourself. Surplus value, in other words.

Note: *Manners are manhood in action, good rehearsal for delivering surplus value.*

STAND UP

When a stranger enters the room, my sons need to rise and acknowledge their arrival. This happened, or didn't happen, recently. Someone showed up late to a sit-down dinner and went around the table shaking everyone's hand. "Get up," I hissed to my youngest, and he did. Later he protested that no one else at the table besides us stood up. I told him this was an excellent observation, but he wasn't everybody else.

Few things are less impressive than a blank-faced kid extending a dead hand to an adult while looking down at the floor or off to one side and in general acting like meeting anyone thirteen or older is time wasted.

Eye contact is nonverbal communication. It's like an emoji or a semicolon, expressing what words don't. It conveys at a minimum interest, sincerity, attentiveness, rapport, and the likelihood of follow-through. In the animal kingdom, it has a link to challenge, and even dominance, whereas failing to make eye contact shows submission.

Don't overdo it—three seconds max. Any longer than that and it comes across as suspicious, hostile, or weird.

ALSO? ASK QUESTIONS

Queen Elizabeth had a favorite line when meeting strangers: *Have you come far?* I remind my boys not to just say hi or hey, confident in the knowledge they're too young and adorable to know better, but to ask follow-up questions, too. People love to talk about themselves—I do—and are flattered by any show of curiosity, even if it's *How long have you lived here?* My boys shouldn't assume everyone is riveted by their adolescent selves. Kick it back, especially if a person is older, which, given the age of my sons, is everybody. *Do you have kids? Where do they go to school? How long have you lived in London?* If none work, try *Have you come far?*

I have work colleagues I loan my New York City loft to, friends who are passing through London, various college and grad school buddies. Dragging a suitcase around all day is exhausting. When a guest shows up, it's good to show them to their room and help set them up.

MEN: PAY FOR WOMEN IF YOU CAN

This one probably sounds sexist, but I don't care. Women may be killing it at work and in higher education, but that doesn't take away from the fact that men still have more economic opportunity and that the gender pay gap exists. So, men, pay for women if you can. Inside all of us is the fear we'll end up alone, friendless, and broke. This fear is more present in women, especially the last. Even if a woman outearns you, your protective instinct should kick in. If you can afford it, pay for meals, also movie and theater tickets, coatrooms, taxis, everything but her car payments. If I could eliminate what my mom lived with, in part on account of my dad's miserliness, I would. Don't be the person he was if you can help it.

American professor/podcast host hit by bus in London/was glancing the wrong way—sometimes I like to imagine what my tombstone might read. I hope the word "generous" shows up somewhere. It probably sounds like virtue signaling, but I enjoy paying for other people. Not because I'm noble, more that as a boy I was so traumatized by my dad's relationship to money. I never want anyone else to go through that.

Having grown up poor in Scotland, my dad brought new meaning to "parsimony." Once he took my best friend Adam and me to go see the movie *Grease*. When the movie ended, he collected two bucks from Adam. I had to sit there watching this shit go down. It was excruciating.

Another time, when I was twelve or thirteen, my dad invited me to go on a big golf vacation in Hawaii—he'd been named ITT Salesperson of the Year or something. Linda came with us. At one point, we went to Baskin-Robbins. My dad and Linda got ice cream, and I ordered a milkshake. For the next forty-eight hours, my dad wouldn't talk to me or look at me. When you're a thirteen-year-old boy who looks up to his father, naturally you wonder what you've done to make him ignore you. Finally, I asked Linda. She told me my dad was upset I'd ordered a milkshake that cost three bucks without clearing it with him first.

When I was at UCLA, I remember thinking, *If I ever make money, I won't be like him. I won't just enjoy having money; I'll share it.* Even today, I can't stand being around cheap people. I know a few rich people who always seem to find a creative reason never to pick up the restaurant bill. I find this grotesque. If my rich friends aren't body-slamming one another to be the first to pay, then we're not friends.

Being generous is one of the best feelings in the world. Last Christmas, my sister Asheley turned fifty—in the Galloway household that means she was turning forty—and I treated her and her family to a trip to South Africa. As the only daughter of my dad and Linda, and ten years younger than me, Asheley and I grew up in separate households. We always got along well but didn't really have a close relationship until I was in my early forties. It was fun waking up to the realization that I, an only child, had an intelligent, interesting, incredibly nice sister I got along with and felt a strong familial bond with. Asheley is fantastic, not to mention a key player in the care and maintenance of our dad as he's aged, and I love hanging out with her. I'm always surprised by the number of siblings I know who not only don't get along but actively hate each other. I hope my two sons remain close, not just for the sake of their mom but also for themselves. Being at a point economically in my life where I can provide Asheley a good memory gave me, a glass-half-empty kind of guy, an amazing amount of joy.

A second arguably sexist idea—a man should always hold a door open for a woman. Take care of others, put them first. Yes, some women will tense, or scowl, implying you're out of touch and need to update your OS, but do it anyway. Always look for where you can add value.

If a new water pitcher arrives at the dinner table, don't fill your glass first. Fill or refill the empty glasses before yours. This one is about you no longer being in a high chair, wearing a bib. Others get served before you serve yourself. Again, think surplus value.

DON'T INTERRUPT

You might be incisive and fascinating, with a grasp of high and low culture, even know the name of that bastard Emily Ratajkowski was photographed leaving that South Beach restaurant with (was his name Scott?). Online culture makes it easy to butt in, burn, and fact-check others in real time. However, wait your turn. Let others finish their thought and listen, rather than simply biding your time to be able to say your piece.

SAY "PLEASE" AND "THANK YOU"

My boys are still young enough so that the presence or absence of manners boomerangs back to their dad and mom. When they get to college, we'll recede, but in the meantime, "pleases" and "thank yous" go a long way.

BE PREPARED

I remember when I saw a step change in my then eleven-year-old. It was wondrous. It was his first week back in school. He left the fourth grade a boy who swore every morning he had unbearable stomach pain—he had to be literally dragged out of bed. But as a new fifth grader, he asked us to help him organize his homework the night before—he wanted "to impress Ms. Jensen."

Hearing this, I told him that a man expresses quiet confidence and that one of the ways you develop quiet confidence is by being prepared, and that I was really impressed with him as he was clearly developing into a man. He beamed . . . I mean beamed. A feeling of reward and confidence visibly washed over him, and he lurched to hug me. Only instead of running into my arms, he evaded my embrace, ran into his older brother's room, hit him in the face, and screamed, "Nobody likes you!" Everyone celebrates in their own way. I told him to stop (being a dad means issuing several million verbal warnings each day) and said he needed to get to bed right away. He responded, as he does dozens of times each day, with "Why?" "Because . . . you have school in the morning."

My older son is at boarding school now—we knew he'd thrive being away from home—and I see good changes in him, too. Sleepaway schools are basically outsourced parenting, but no one can accuse them of doing a bad job. When he comes home on the weekends, he's kinder, more polite and disciplined—better man . . . ners, in short. Both my boys make me so proud.

Manners are the escutcheon of a man who knows who he is. Practice them so they become as unthinking as tying your sneakers or answering in monosyllables when your dad asks you about your day. They give you a head start in creating surplus value, help you make friends, get women, get hired at work, and become a role model and a generally impressive human being.

chapter 10

LIFE IS SO RICH

THE TAO OF ENOUGH

I always had issues with *enough*, was always dissatisfied. I wanted more, and after that ... *more*.

The impulse to want more is instinctual and healthy. You are what you settle for, Janis Joplin (not making this up) said. The problem comes when you don't enjoy what you have while you have it. It took me a while to learn how to enjoy what I had, to be present in the moment. Instead I was in the rat race to prove myself. At first my thirst for more was motivating. It gave me confidence, pushed me to take risks. Then I assigned myself a number that kept increasing as time passed. I reached a point where I had enough money to take care of my mom and help with other family members. Should have been enough, but it wasn't.

In the 1970s, the capitalist equation was simple. My dad's boss had a slightly nicer car and an exponentially bigger house than ours. But people of all incomes showed up at the same church and country club. There wasn't the delta that exists today, based on the market's ability to sanctify superior experiences based on incremental amounts of money, where we rarely spend time with people outside our own ecosystems.

My own equation seemed simple. At some point, I had enough money to fly business class and live in a nice house. Done. That should have been it, except I didn't stop the bullshit. My *more* addiction grew: Why live in Westwood when Beverly Hills is nearby? How about a vacation house in Aspen? I went from wanting to own a million-dollar house to coveting a $30 million mountaintop property. Fuck business class, too—what about flying private? Sure, now and then I chartered a private plane for special events, but . . . hold on . . . I now want . . . to fly private . . . all the time. I bought a Challenger 300. Owning a plane is like managing a business—too much work. A Gulfstream was within reach—so I bought a quarter share. In sum, the appreciation and gratitude I felt once stretching out in Delta business class evolved into me contemplating, unironically, a $65 million jet.

Why not try to be a billionaire? I would start a private equity fund with my own money and raise the rest. I was rounding third, had good contacts, and a feel for the market. Finding some cool companies to invest in or take private would be easy. Two phone calls later, I had raised $50 million.

Then that year I lost two good friends: Scott (another Scott) and Craig. Scott was my good friend and New York City drinking buddy. It happened fast—a head bump, a diagnosis of mild leukemia, chemo that worked and then didn't, a stem cell transplant from his son, improvement, hope, relapse. He was buried a month later. Craig, my first-year roommate at UCLA, was another fit, handsome guy. He got Guillain-Barré syndrome, where the immune system attacks the nerves. It's rare and incurable. His arms and legs swelled, he went in for a test—and his heart stopped. Scott and Craig were both healthy, wonderful guys.

Their loss really hit me. My grief taught me that I wouldn't be around much longer myself. Did I want to get back on that wheel, working long days managing other people's money and buying companies?

I'm the opposite of a workaholic—I'm outstanding at not working. Time was passing. I called the investors back, canceled the fund idea. *This is it*, I thought. *This is enough*. I still had money fears, mostly about me doing something stupid in a recession and losing everything, but I also didn't want those fears to drive my entire life. Mostly I loved—still do—spending time with my wife and kids and dogs, traveling, doing fun, crazy things. Frida Kahlo said, *I want my death to be glorious, and I don't want to come back*. Right now, I'm dying—everyone is—and I hope my own departure is glorious and binding.

Putting myself there, at near death, helps me sort through life and weigh decisions that provide peace. I know at the end I'll be more upset about the risks I didn't take than about the fallout from the ones I did. I'll feel joy that I kissed my boys every day, let my dogs up onto the couch, and dressed up as Elizabeth Holmes on CNN+. I would've been angry had I kept being so angry so much, upset had I stayed addicted to *more*, and been disappointed if I'd let fear, or my need for people's approval, get in the way of living out loud.

STUFF AND NONSENSE

If you're over fifty, marketers (except Cologuard) treat you like a kid hobbling around on crutches at the school prom. Show me a company with operating margins north of 30 percent, and I'll show you a business that's either tapped into addiction or the young, irrational mating mind. In my thirties, I had a Panerai watch, drove a BMW with special wheels, and evinced a strange willingness to spend $450 on a bottle of Grey Goose at a nightclub. These objects signaled in all caps my value as a mate so I could attract an evolutionarily superior female.

In marketing, eighteen-to-twenty-five-year-olds set the tone for trends/style/fashion—but businesses and brands mostly focus on twenty-five- to fifty-four-year-olds; i.e., irrational idiots willing to part with money to increase their chances of reproductive success.

Age makes you more rational. People fifty-plus know that a new sweater or pair of $400 headphones won't transform them or offer transcendence. A time horizon looms. What matters are healthcare, grandkids, savoring moments, and freaking out about retirement, longevity, and end-of-life health costs.

I have a talent for spending stupid money on all varieties of ridiculous shit. I deny myself nothing, though I'm not into *stuff*. I find peace in order, simplicity, no clutter. I don't even own a car. We recently moved, and I threw out or donated three-quarters of everything I owned. I have two sets of clothes, one for working out, another for work. Four out of five days, I wear the same uniform: Tommy John underwear, Bombas socks, Rag & Bone pants, a James Perse shirt, and Warby Parker glasses. Saves thinking and time.

Instead of buying things, my money goes toward experiences and real estate, the former a strategy making it impossible for my sons to avoid me. In twenty years, if they can put up with a meal with dad, they can spend the rest of the vacation skiing or swimming or drinking.

Last year, I took Nolan to see the Paris Saint-Germain football team play in Paris. We took the Eurostar. After checking into our hotel, we went out for our favorite meal, steak frites. I took a nap. Nolan went for a swim in the pool. We had an amazing dinner that night and then went to the stadium. It was raining. PSG lost. Returning to the hotel, we slept, woke up, had more incredible food for breakfast, and got on the Eurostar back to London.

It was an insane plan, also a fantastic way to spend time with my son, one that surpassed anything my fantasy life could have come up with. My son and I taking the Eurostar to Paris for forty-eight hours together was all that mattered. There was no more—this was enough.

A SMALL GOOD THING

If cashmere and headphones lose their reproductive appeal over time, what replaces them? Small things, mini-moments. I find beauty and joy and grace in little, amazing moments that I would have once been too busy and distracted to notice.

In Paris, Nolan and I visited a few stores near our hotel. One sold the most beautiful candles I'd ever seen. It hit me—someone, somewhere, got really good at making candles and now devotes their life to creating exquisite configurations of colored burning wax. I found this inspiring. Next door was a chocolatier with exquisite truffles, pralines, and ganaches behind glass. I was inspired all over again. At the PSG game, crowds of fairly conventional-looking men were jumping up and down, beating drums in forty-degree wet weather. It was a fantastic sight, again inspiring. Before boarding the Eurostar, we went inside Notre Dame, which had just reopened. I've never cared about religious institutions, but one glance at the stained glass made me think humans are onto something good.

Sometimes I listen to old B-52 songs—I used to dance to them. John Lennon loved the band; their example helped convince him to do *Double Fantasy* with Yoko Ono. How, though, did five weirdos from the University of Georgia in Athens have the confidence to write, "Has anyone seen a dog dyed dark green?" or "You're living underground like a wild potato" and believe they might earn a living someday? That American society is impressive and secure enough to encourage the eccentric among us inspires me, too. So does the courage and creativity required to write about rock lobsters. A founding member, Ricky Wilson, died of AIDS in the eighties. He was thirty-two and kept the disease secret. Once my response would have been rueful, remote—*Wow, AIDS, awful*. These days it hits me in the gut. I think about his parents, and what if better AIDS meds had been available back then: Could he have gone on to a career like John Lennon's?

Aging is a double-edged sword. The good news is you get more thoughtful. The bad news is you get more thoughtful. Time starts falling off a cliff; you begin barreling toward the end. A friend or two, men and women you love, die. New injuries and ailments remind you, *Shit, I'm actually mortal, I'm going to die*. You never believe it when you're a kid. You see the beauty and the tragedy of life in 4K. The mundane pops, the quotidian sings. Outside my house in Florida is a beautiful bright-red bougainvillea. It's extraordinary. I may live in London, but I think about it every day, like a child. There will come a time when I go swimming in the ocean for the last time; doing the math, I have thirty to fifty swims left in me, and fewer visits to Paris. Pondering all this, mortality, both its joy and fear, is upsetting, overwhelming, and beautiful.

FAME

Until my forties, I was known: known in grad school at Berkeley, known in the e-commerce scene in the Bay Area, and, after having taught five thousand students, known around NYU's campus. Then, in 2016, the team at L2, my business intelligence firm, was headed to our weekly team lunch when, from across the street, we heard, "Prof G! We love your videos!" Two Indian men in their twenties hurriedly crossed the street to tell me they never missed our *Winners & Losers* videos and that I had a following in India. Then they asked for a selfie. The whole team found it odd and amusing that people from several thousand miles away not only knew our work, but also felt affection and admiration for it.

My recognition has grown since. Tourists from Michigan ran out of a restaurant recently to ask if I could wait a minute while they, proud moms, got their (horrified) sons to take a selfie with me: "We listen to your pod together." And I receive dozens of emails and hundreds of comments from people I've never met or been in the same room with. I love being recognized. As a bit of a megalomaniac, I can't think of a time when it didn't make me feel good, even if I was in a hurry. People are so wonderful to me, it (almost) convinces me that we're having an impact. A study shows that one in ten Americans say fame is important to them. I'm the one.

There are dark linings to the silver cloud. The allure of fame takes some people to dark places, so it matters where the void that people try and fill with fame comes from. For me, I believe the void is that, growing up, I was invisible. Not a good or bad student, neither a loner nor especially social, athletic but not talented, funny but not hilarious. At big public schools, it was pretty easy to blend into the ecosystem as a defense mechanism against predators who were more popular, mean, or even violent. An especially bad acne week? Rejection from a person/group beyond my social reach? No problem, just retreat and become invisible. Loved by my mom at home, I was also less visible to my dad, and trying so hard to be seen.

So my limited fame fills a hole, an old fear that I'd never amount to anything. I'd remain invisible and . . . alone. A hole leaks, though, so it never fills up. Recognition from strangers, as you age, feels increasingly like empty calories. The affection people have for you is for your public avatar—it's not really for you, as they don't know you. And if they did, they'd likely be disappointed. I understand why truly famous, A-list people feel they can't leave the house. At the same time, I don't understand people who complain about fame. If it's a function of their work: just stop working and shut up for a few months; you'll be amazed how fast the culture moves on.

Still, the saving grace is that, in person, people are wonderful, and my limited amount of fame is for things people generally appreciate (I'm not Pol Pot or Jeffrey Epstein). Online, significantly less so. A nonzero percentage of online recognition is really ugly. The inevitable corollary of success is that people feel the need to take you down, and online media has tapped into that instinct like nothing else. There seems to be a cottage industry for correcting or calling people out once they have (any) fame. I'd like to say it just rolls off of me, but it doesn't. Some of it is downright disturbing. Recently, I've been receiving emails from (purportedly) young men experiencing suicidal ideation who need help (i.e., money) with pleads closely tailored to my publicly stated views and the concerns of this book. They're clearly fakes (possibly AI-generated) but still disturbing. Fame has validated for me what almost every study shows: anything that happens in real life is profoundly better, kinder, and more human than its online facsimile. And I'm not even that famous.

Fame and atheism go well together because the only thing that survives death is living people's memory of you and if it influences their actions. A few decades from now, I'll be gone. When I think about that (which is often), I am reminded that I don't need the recognition of strangers to make me immortal. There are two men who lived with me the first eighteen-plus years of their lives who will remember me. They'll remember how intense, yet goofy, I was. I'd also like to believe they'll be more kind and secure than I was, as every day their dad confirmed they were wonderful and immensely loved. They won't remember my books or podcasts, the TV networks I helped kill, or any other accomplishments. They will feel me, though. They'll tell stories about me; I'm certain of it. I'll be famous.

LOSING MY RELIGION

My religious indoctrination growing up was more varied than consistent. When I was at my dad's, I'd go with Linda to a Unitarian church. At my mom's, we'd go intermittently to temple.

While inconsistent, the impact of religion on my development was real. I remember the rabbi at Temple Isaiah delivering a *d'var Torah* that spanned from the conflict in the Middle East to the role of friendship. Afterward, over a brisket dip at Junior's Deli, my mom and I discussed the sermon, and I remember thinking, *This is fun, and I'm good at it* (meaning Judaism). I asked my mom what rabbis did and how much money they made. "They educate and comfort people, and not much. However, they command a great deal of respect."

In high school, my closest friend, Brett, was Mormon. He was part of a two-parent family who loved sports, laughed a lot, and treated me well. As a latchkey kid, I was at the Jarvis household almost every day. I went to church events, played on Mormon sports teams, and even went to services a few times, though I never felt any pressure to sign up.

My path to atheism has been downhill. I've always been skeptical and judgmental. I consider myself a scientist. Without fail, when an elected official in the United States begins referencing the Bible or talking about Jesus, he's about to advocate for cutting food stamps to single mothers. If Jesus, as dozens of congresspeople believe, does return, I believe he will show up in many of their offices and vomit on them. Religion is easy to poke holes in and contrary to academia. I've come to esteem the role religious institutions play in society and people's lives. The voyage began with my being curious about religion, then not understanding it, which led to intellectual disdain—*An invisible friend, huh?*—and is ending with respect and humility. For most people, religion is a source of comfort, community, and compassion. Seneca believed religion was regarded by the poor as true, the wise as false, and the powerful as useful. But I find the absence of religion and opportunities to congregate with strangers leaves a void. I'm getting older, wanting to serve in the agency of others, to be part of something bigger, and register comfort. I do this with my family and the young men I mentor. Is that enough?

Atheism is a belief, too. In the same way it's my right to not believe in God, I also have an obligation to believe in the rights of other people to have a God. I'd also like to think that the absence of preordained truths fosters a relentless pursuit of knowledge, a deeper appreciation for the wonders of the universe, and a profound respect for the inherent value of all living beings.

At some point, I will look into my sons' eyes and know our relationship is coming to an end. That knowledge puts me squarely in the moment. It's given me a strong appreciation of the finite nature of life and how under no circumstances is this a dress rehearsal. I've become kinder, more present, more out there with my emotions.

More than anything, this serves as a combatant against fear. What I worry about—mostly what other people think about me—is dumb. Those people will be dead soon, and I will, too. I find this more liberating than depressing.

There are moments when I feel that there is something other than just us humans. Less "bigger," maybe, than beyond understanding. My bet is that slowly, surely, science will get to the bottom of it. Believing there's nothing conscious or sentient in the afterlife has helped me be more generous, more loving, and more spiritual while I'm here. It's a belief system of sorts focused on the now. If there are no rewards for leading a virtuous life, it's made me better appreciate the role virtue plays in this one.

Lacking grace as a young man, I think I would have benefited from more time in religious institutions. When I got ketamine therapy, the medical director came into the room before injecting me, asked everyone to put out their hands, and said, *Let's pray*. One or two decades ago, the assumption that I was religious would have bugged me (then again, we were in Texas). Now I thought, *This is really nice, just being in the company of strangers, holding hands, wishing one another the best*. There was no downside whatsoever.

LONG GOODBYE

My dad is dying.

One of my greatest sources of pride was giving my mom a good death. I've virtue signaled about it before. My dad is at that stage, and it's time for me to step in and be the generous, loving person I'd like to think I am.

But I haven't. The love I gave my mom sprung from the love I have for her and the love she gave me from day one. Up late at night, calming me with math problems as my nosebleed would not cauterize for hours. Honking the horn, after a ten-hour-day at the secretarial pool she managed, as she drove into the garage of our apartment complex, to then spend more hours teaching me how to drive stick in her lime-green Opel Manta.

As Suze Orman says, small regular investments/savings at a young age have immense payoff when you're older. Compound interest holds true in relationships. The mothers, fathers, aunts, uncles, mentors, and strangers who invest in you early warrant immense returns decades later. My father wasn't a bad father, but he left us, and even when he was there, it was fraught. However, my dad is a much better father to me than his dad was to him—his father beat him. He was a better father to my younger sister (granted, she's more likable), and as he grew older, he's been a better father to me. The efforts he made and didn't make still resonate and inspire my sister and me to be better parents to our children.

Our relationship with our parents is complicated. However, near the end things get simpler. When he's gone, I will miss him a great deal. And while here, he's better than what he came from. He inspires me to be the same.

Life isn't about what happens to you—it's about how you respond to it.

GIVING BACK

At a certain point, there's no reason why anyone should have over a certain amount of wealth.

Since I find that money is a scorecard, making it hard to stop pursuing more, I've imposed a tax on myself. Every year, I give away more than I spend. I sit down, calculate how much I've paid out, and aim to give away twice that to people in need, nonprofits, higher ed, charities focused on vocational programs and mental health. Almost every week I give away money—random amounts, too, from $1K to ten grand—to individuals who I sense could use it. This is virtue signaling (again) but so what. It makes me feel patriotic. It's fun. I get a rush. I feel good about myself. It makes me feel masculine.

Until the age of forty-five, I was the least philanthropic person in the world. The money I made I banked. I lived high on the hog, was never disciplined about saving, lacked character, and gave nothing away. Until I was financially bulletproof, I put myself first. I didn't do anything for anybody or give money to anyone unless it could benefit me.

But then I reached a certain point of economic security that gave me enough room to reassess. I realized I had been living in fear of not having money and coping with scarcity. I told myself that, from then on, any even incrementally extra amount of money I made I would give away. Giving in the agency of something bigger than myself makes me feel good. Is what I do now generous? Not really. While I give big numbers away, it has almost no impact on my life. If I gave away half, it could. In a capitalist society, I want to provide financial security for my family. But men (and women) can continue to explore how to provide and protect so their families are safe while offering more to their communities and country. How do we provide surplus value, financially and well beyond?

I wish I hadn't waited as long as I did. I would argue that anyone who starts giving away money at a young age finds it compounds. You feel good about yourself. Others respect you. It's another form of surplus value. You're giving back what life, schools, churches, your parents, and other adults have provided you. Some people never reach a point of surplus value. They keep taking—from their friends, their parents, their siblings, their partners, the government. The goal as always is to give more than you take in—resources, love, kindness, understanding, friendship, or whatever else—while generating more of those things for others.

Before I die, I want to make damn sure that in that dimension I'm in the black. That I provide more love to my sons than my own parents gave me, and my mom provided *a lot* for me. That's the basis of human evolution. Do better. Love people more. Be a better friend, employer. Give back what you got, times a hundred.

TEARING UP

Crying may have an evolutionary purpose, as it signals surrender (*Please stop what you are doing to me*), elicits empathy from those around you, and can help parents locate their offspring. For babies, active crying may be a way of restoring equilibrium after overstimulation. One way to solve this is to mimic the womb with the five-S's method—Swaddle, Side-stomach position, Shush, Swing, Suck—developed by Dr. Harvey Karp. (That shit is genius.)

Crying can also relieve the stress brought on by an onslaught of emotions that are difficult to process. I grew up with the message that men aren't supposed to cry, which likely is a function of the whole surrender thing.

The first time I remember crying, I mean really crying, was at age nine. My mom had left my dad and me solo. I was watching, on a Friday night at eight thirty, pre-DVR, *The Partridge Family* with my dad. We were sitting on the couch in matching orange terry cloth robes, the height of opulence in 1970s middle-class America. My dad had received these luxury items as swag for playing in a golf tournament hosted by his firm. He snagged a size small for me, which was still eight sizes too big for a nine-year-old.

Embroidered on the chest of our Tang-colored slouchwear was a red flagstick above green cursive that read *Pebble Beach*. I didn't know where Pebble Beach was, but I knew important people played golf there, which meant my dad was important. I had not yet registered the reality of my parents' divorce, but it suddenly came to me, and so, draped in my Turkish cotton tent, I began to sob uncontrollably. I cried for a good thirty minutes. My dad seemed panicked and kept saying, "I'm so sorry, is there anything I can do?" I would respond "No, I'm just sad." That was our first real conversation.

Between ages thirty-four and forty-four, I lost the capacity to cry. Didn't cry when I got divorced or when my mom died. It felt like I just forgot how. I was self-numbing by being obsessed with business and became hugely stressed over it. Avoiding my feelings and deeper emotional life, I wrapped way too much of my identity and self-worth around professional success. But I never cried because of business. And, trust me, there have been good reasons several (hundred) times.

However, since my mid-forties, something strange has happened: I. Cry. All. The. Time.

Pretty sure it's a good thing. Sorrowful crying is looking to the past with sadness or to the future with dread; it helps me grieve the past and be more in the present. Crying as a result of happiness is a response to a moment as if it's eternal; the person is frozen in a blissful, immortalized present. My tears lately have been the latter as I slow down and pursue moments. Moments with friends, moments trying to freeze time with my kids, and (mostly) just feeling very in the moment. Something about being on a plane turns me into a mess. Anytime I talk about my mom or sons or watch a movie or TV show involving a parent-child relationship, especially mom-son, my voice starts cracking. I also choke up in class more often, in front of 120 kids in their late twenties. I used to feel embarrassed and tell myself I need to keep it together. But as we get older we become more like ourselves, and I'm getting more comfortable with raw emotions, and if there's potential collateral damage, I've earned it.

As you get older and begin to register the finite time we have, you want to slow time and have moments when you feel the beauty around and in you. Depression isn't feeling sad but feeling nothing. Crying—especially in the company of, or thinking about, loved ones—feels healthy and joyous. I well up thinking about it.

THANKS, I'LL PASS

Last weekend I went to a wonderful funeral. I never met the deceased but went since I know his (grown) kids. The funeral home couldn't fit all the people who showed up, so we were stuck in the back, couldn't see anything, and listened to the eulogies over a poor PA system. The words were moving. There was the lifelong friend serving as MC who struck exactly the right tone and quoted from (no joke) Dr. Seuss:

"Don't cry because it's over, smile because it happened."

Every eulogy contained rich examples of how much the man had loved life, as evidenced by his generosity and passion for a good time. There was the decades-long colleague who referenced the skills and formidable success his mentor registered and, at the end of his eulogy, paused, broke down, and proclaimed, "He was like a father to me, and I loved him." I think that may be the nicest thing anybody can say about someone else.

Central to the prosperity and survival of our species is mothers and fathers who have an irrational passion for their kids' well-being. To fill this role for people who aren't your offspring is generosity toward the planet and species. I've never understood the idolatry of Steve Jobs. The world needs more engaged fathers, not a better fucking phone.

The deceased's kids are living testaments to what a great person he was. They both share a comedy gene—two of the funniest people any of us know. Their humor stems from the confidence to be outrageous, an ability to see irony in almost everything, and joy at seeing others laugh and have a good time. These qualities are likely a result of warm, loving, and generous parents. Methinks that would be a decent tombstone.

The service was what I imagine most of us want, if a long time from now: a standing-room-only crowd of people who are crying because it's over but can't help smiling because it happened.

I can see my death. I was twenty-five yesterday, and I'll be eighty-four tomorrow. I can imagine the people, photos, music, and drugs I want to have around me, and even feel my thoughts at that moment. I've set money aside. I want people I love around me. I want to fall asleep in a really comfortable bed. I daresay it will be amazing. I can't say I look forward to it, but I dread it less.

Reminder: this is as good as it gets. And it's magnificent. I hate my life less and less every day.

CONCLUSION

A Letter to My Sons

Alec and Nolan,

I write this book inspired by you. I love both of you so much and am incredibly proud of you. You're becoming impressive young men and good citizens. Being your dad has been the most meaningful experience in my life.

If/when you read this book, I hope it resonates. As you have been growing up, I've witnessed a crisis with the boys and young men just ahead of you. It alarms me. And as a protector, I want to do something—reach back into my own story, review research, offer advice about your journeys and how you travel these paths.

We are mammals, and mammals thrive in packs/herds/schools, etc. Try to limit the amount of time you spend alone. This won't be easy, as the deepest-pocketed firms with the most talented people, armed with godlike technology, will try to convince you that you can have a low-friction, easier version of life on a screen with an algorithm. You need to be around other people, as much as possible. Go into the office, join organizations, say yes to nearly any invitation, and make plans with others.

Colleagues, friends, romantic partners, and family are the key to happiness and, along the way, provide the discipline, learning, and guardrails we all need to develop into the best versions of ourselves. An enemy of masculinity is isolation. "He's so impressive and spends so much time alone," said no one ever.

Everybody needs downtime, and maybe you'll get strength from meditation and mindfulness. However, greatness is in the agency of others and you should have roommates, go into the office, spend time with mates, ask people out, and participate in as many collectives as possible—concerts, events, movies, etc.

"Protector" is the sturdiest of the three legs of what it means to be male. Take it seriously as a good citizen, friend, husband, and father. The reality is a lot of your blessings are just that . . . blessings—not your doing. You were born into a democracy and money, which have provided, thus far, an extraordinary life. This comes at a price, specifically a debt. You have an obligation to protect and advocate for others, because you were born with advantages others don't have. Alec and I just finished a college tour of some of the most elite universities, and Nolan just returned from a field trip to the beaches of Normandy. These experiences set you apart from many others, including what I or my parents could experience at your age. I am the first person, on either side of our family, to graduate from high school.

I hope you are real patriots and support and defend your country (America). Four of your most formative years were spent in the UK, which has been wonderful for all of us. But this experience was afforded to us because of the opportunities and prosperity your parents recognized in America. Your parents would have never registered similar opportunities had we lived somewhere else. I hope you will continue our support of the nation that gave us so much. Vote, pay taxes, and be an evangelist for our nation and its values. Also, try to give people the benefit of the doubt and treat them with respect, if for no other reason because they are fellow Americans.

Women can gestate bones, organs, and then give birth. This is singular. As men, you are blessed with denser bone structure, more muscle mass, and testosterone that can be turned into incredible physical strength. Embrace this blessing. Your grandfather got me working out when I was twelve, and I've done the same for you. Try to get, and stay, really strong. You'll be happier, kinder, and more attractive. And with this size and strength, protect others, whether opening doors, helping people get their suitcase off a baggage carousel, or breaking up fights.

Remember to be kind to others, and to yourselves. Like golf or piano, kindness is a practice. This was a big lesson for me because when I was your age, I wasn't kind. Not mean, just not kind. As I got older, I made an effort to practice small acts of kindness until it became second nature. It's a life hack hiding in plain sight as people notice, and it will put you in a room of opportunities.

Try to be more emotive—reckless even—with your emotions, with your concern, hurt, sadness, and admiration, especially with your family and friends. It's what informs your life, knowing what's important to you and inspires you. From the age of twenty-nine to forty-four, I didn't cry or laugh out loud much. I see these years as mostly wasted as I was sleepwalking through life, barely conscious. I don't want this for you. We have great advantages as a species, like our brain, opposable thumbs, willingness to cooperate, and a broader range of emotions. Use them.

Your goal is to provide surplus value, to offer more than you're given without keeping score. Work to be able to absorb the chaos and anxiety around you without it absorbing you; take arrows; be an active and big part of your loved ones' lives; and never lose sight of your role as protector. The most masculine people leave a legacy of surplus value from a place of kindness, generosity, and strength. They give more love, hope, and encouragement, pay more taxes, and create more jobs than they get back.

Think of the most masculine jobs, including firefighters and the armed forces. Those men (and women) signal discipline, order, confidence, and patriotism, and have a code; i.e., they know who they are and what to do. Part of becoming a man is acting as if you are wearing military fatigues, recognizing that a core reason you are here is to protect yourself, your partner, your family, and your country.

It's not just physical. Shit-posting or criticizing another person or group behind their back isn't protection; it's anti-masculine. Either step up to defend others or keep quiet. You may not share the values of every community. But if you see any community, no matter which one, getting demonized by politicians or railed against by anonymous social media accounts, your instinct should be to protect first.

I hope you embrace your strength, physical and mental, as you go forward. That you take risks, whether it's applying to colleges you're unqualified for or approaching someone you're attracted to who is out of your league. The world is not yours for the taking but the trying. Try really hard. Your dad's success was that I was never afraid to punch above my weight. Fear of (public) failure is an enemy of masculinity. If you're not failing, you're not progressing.

I hope you two will grow up to be better friends. I can't force it. Siblings are meant to be annoying. They also understand you better than almost anyone else. But, as a nod to me, I hope you give each other the benefit of the doubt and make an effort to be close.

I am fifteen years older than your mother, so she'll likely be around long after I'm gone. I demand, once I'm gone, that you love and support and cooperate to take care of your mother. You'll move out, meet your own mates, be juggling demands on yourselves and your time. But please come together—show up—and continue to love and take care of your mom.

Be cognizant of bad habits and ways of numbing out that get in the way of living a full life. Whether too much alcohol, gambling, food, drugs, porn, or laziness, try to course-correct, and if it's difficult to address, get help. Ask for help. Not enough men do this. Don't go online for answers; find a person.

Let yourself be happy. Be less hard on yourself than I was on myself. I've wasted years and joy focused on what I missed or screwed up versus my blessings and accomplishments. Learn from what I did wrong. Be me + better.

And, as a favor to me, try to evolve our family DNA and do something I've struggled with: acknowledge and embrace the moments of your life as you experience them. It's the only thing we really have: the here, the now.

I'll finish where I started: I love you immensely. It is impossible (now) for you to grasp how I feel about you. Impossible, but soon . . . obvious. When? When you have a son.

And, again . . . take care of your mom.

Dad

Acknowledgments

Putting this book together was so uncharacteristically stress-free, it was worrisome. My agent, Jim Levine, provided early counsel and keen direction. My editor, Stephanie Frerich, kept the work on and on schedule, as did her boss, Jon Karp.

My colleague and partner at ProfG Media, Katherine Dillon, is steady and steadying—it's impossible to imagine life without her. Peter Smith, our writer, spent months turning my chicken shit into chicken salad. Peter is the most talented writer I have worked with, and this book could not have happened without him. Lily Smith tackled the citations with aplomb and discipline. Lastly, I'm indebted to Richard Reeves, our Yoda on this topic, whose work and passion continue to inspire me.

Notes

INTRODUCTION

2 *First, boys face*: Adrianne Frech et al., "The Myth of Men's Stable, Continuous Labor Force Attachment: Multitrajectories of U.S. Baby Boomer Men's Employment," *Socius* 9 (2023): 1–27, https://doi.org/10.1177/23780231231197031.

2 *Many grow up without*: Richard Reeves, "Missing Misters: Gender Diversity Among Teachers," American Institute for Boys and Men, February 27, 2024, https://aibm.org/research/missing-misters/.

2 *A prohibitive real estate market*: Reeves, "Missing Misters."

3 *The percentage of young men*: Mona Lazar, "Young Men Are Failing and Taking Society Down with Them," Medium, January 13, 2025, https://medium.com/fourth-wave/young-men-are-failing-and-taking-society-down-with-them-fbb8ce20ea52.

3 *Workforce participation among men*: Lazar, "Young Men Are Failing."

3 *From 2005 to 2019*: Carol Graham, "America's Crisis of Despair: A Federal Task Force for Economic Recovery and Societal Well-Being," Brookings Institution, July 2021, https://www.brookings.edu/articles/americas-crisis-of-despair-a-federal-task-force-for-economic-recovery-and-societal-well-being/.

3 *Excluding deaths caused*: Joint Economic Committee, "Long-Term Trends in Deaths of Despair," September 5, 2019, https://www.jec.senate.gov/public/index.cfm/republicans/2019/9/long-term-trends-in-deaths-of-despair.

3 *Today, hypogamy*: Stephanie H. Murray, "The New Marriage of Unequals," *Atlantic*, March 31, 2025, https://www.theatlantic.com/family/archive/2025/03/marrying-down-wife-education-hypogamy/682223/.

4 *Here's a terrifying stat*: Dean Brooks, "45% of Men Age 18–25 Have Never Approached a Woman in Person," Medium, August 2024, https://dean

maxbrooks.medium.com/45-of-men-age-18-25-have-never-approached-a-woman-in-person-087519be4e6b.

5 *The Empire State Building*: American Society of Civil Engineers Metropolitan Section, "Empire State Building," ASCE Metropolitan Section, https://www.ascemetsection.org/committees/history-and-heritage/landmarks/empire-state-building.

5 *The fighting went on*: "Battle of the Bulge Memorial," Arlington National Cemetery, https://www.arlingtoncemetery.mil/Explore/Monuments-and-Memorials/Battle-of-the-Bulge.

6 *It's why, historically and globally*: Ian Sample, "More Women Than Men Have Added Their DNA to the Human Gene Pool," *Guardian*, September 24, 2014, https://www.theguardian.com/science/2014/sep/24/women-men-dna-human-gene-pool.

8 *Donald Trump gained 16 percent*: Maryann Cousens, "2024 Post-Election Survey: Gender and Age Analysis of 2024 Election Results," *Navigator*, December 12, 2024, https://navigatorresearch.org/2024-post-election-survey-gender-and-age-analysis-of-2024-election-results/.

1 – BOYHOOD

16 *Along with determining male physiology*: Carole Hooven, *T: The Story of Testosterone* (New York: Henry Holt, 2021), 13.
16 *The role testosterone plays*: Hooven, *T*, 73.
16 *Everyone is born*: Hooven, *T*, 54.
17 *T peaks at age twenty*: Hooven, *T*, 116.
17 *From a young age*: David J. Handelsman, Angelica L. Hirschberg, and Stéphane Bermon, "Circulating Testosterone as the Hormonal Basis of Sex Differences in Athletic Performance," *Endocrine Reviews* 39, no. 5 (October 1, 2018): 803–29, https://doi.org/10.1210/er.2018-00020.
17 *Ultimately, T has one role*: Handelsman, Hirschberg, and Bermon, "Circulating Testosterone," 814.
32 *The male amygdala*: Louann Brizendine, *The Female Brain* (New York: Harmony Books, 2007), 5.
32 *contains testosterone receptors*: Brizendine, *The Female Brain*, 129.
32 *Girls attain "peak values"*: Rhoshel K. Lenroot and Jay N. Giedd, "Sex Differences in the Adolescent Brain," *Brain and Cognition* 72, no. 1 (February 2010): 46–55, https://doi.org/10.1016/j.bandc.2009.10.008.
32 *Basically, the female PFC matures*: "Female Brain Versus Male Brain," *NeuroRelay*, October 7, 2012, http://neurorelay.com/2012/10/07/female-brain-versus-male-brain/.

33 *Their socializing*: Brizendine, *The Female Brain*, 39.

33 *By fourteen to fifteen, girls have*: "Sex Differences in Brain Anatomy," *NIH Research Matters*, February 22, 2021, https://www.nih.gov/news-events/nih-research-matters/sex-differences-brain-anatomy.

33 *Note: diagnostic bias*: Angela Byars-Winston and Maria Lund Dahlberg, eds., National Academies of Sciences, Engineering, and Medicine, *The Science of Effective Mentorship in STEMM* (Washington, DC: The National Academies Press, 2020), https://www.ncbi.nlm.nih.gov/sites/books/NBK606330/.

33 *white kids from higher socioeconomic*: Christina D. Kang-Yi et al., "Racial-Ethnic Disparities in Autism Spectrum Disorder Diagnosis," *Journal of Developmental and Behavioral Pediatrics* 42, no. 8 (October/November 2021): 682–89, https://doi.org/10.1097/DBP.0000000000000996.

34 *As to whether the absence*: Richard V. Reeves, "Missing Misters: Gender Diversity Among Teachers," *American Institute for Boys and Men*, February 27, 2024, https://aibm.org/research/missing-misters/.

34 *Children today are overprotected*: Jonathan Haidt, "The Real Threat to Gen Z Isn't Smartphones. It's the Internet," *New York Times*, March 18, 2024, https://www.nytimes.com/2024/03/18/opinion/internet-kids-social-media.html.

2 – THINGS GET HAIRY: ADOLESCENCE

37 *One study reported that 10 to 30 percent*: D. A. Frederick et al., "Surveys and the Eidemiology of Body Image Dissatisfaction," *Encyclopedia of Body Image and Human Appearance* (2012): 766–74, https://www.sciencedirect.com/science/article/abs/pii/B9780123849250001218.

42 *In 1997, approximately 90 percent*: Shannon Osaka, "'I'll Call an Uber or 911': Why Gen Z Doesn't Want to Drive," *Washington Post*, February 13, 2023, https://www.washingtonpost.com/climate-solutions/2023/02/13/gen-z-driving-less-uber/.

45 *In 2019, 28 percent of Black men*: Richard V. Reeves, Sarah Nzau, and Ember Smith, "The Challenges Facing Black Men—and the Case for Action," Brookings Institution, November 19, 2020, https://www.brookings.edu/articles/the-challenges-facing-black-men-and-the-case-for-action/.

45 *Black workers of both genders*: Michelle Holder, "The 'Double Gap' and the Bottom Line: African American Women's Wage Gap and Corporate Profits," Roosevelt Institute, March 31, 2020, https://rooseveltinstitute.org/publications/the-double-gap-and-the-bottom-line-african-american-womens-wage-gap-and-corporate-profits/.

45 *labor force participation*: U.S. Bureau of Labor Statistics, "Labor Force Participation Rate—20 Yrs. & Over, Black or African American Men," *FRED*, Federal Reserve Bank of St. Louis, accessed April 21, 2025, https://fred.stlouisfed.org/series/LNS11300031.

45 *As of 2021, Black youth*: Joshua Rovner, "Black Disparities in Youth Incarceration," The Sentencing Project, December 12, 2023, https://www.sentencingproject.org/fact-sheet/black-disparities-in-youth-incarceration/.

45 *as of 2010, Black men*: National Research Council, *The Growth of Incarceration in the United States: Exploring Causes and Consequences* (Washington, DC: The National Academies Press, 2014), https://nap.nationalacademies.org/read/18613/chapter/2.

48 *Number three is kindness*: Joao Francisco Goes Braga Takayanagi et al., "What Do Different People Look for in a Partner? Effects of Sex, Sexual Orientation, and Mating Strategies on Partner Preferences," *Archives of Sexual Behavior* 53 (2024): 981–1000, https://doi.org/10.1007/s10508-023-02767-4.

58 *Kids who live in low-income*: Gary W. Evans et al., "Childhood Poverty and Late Adolescents' Blood Pressure Reactivity and Recovery to Acute Stress," *Psychological Science* 24, no. 11 (2013): 2284–91, https://www.ncbi.nlm.nih.gov/pmc/articles/PMC3769521/.

3 — HIGHER EDUCATION

71 *"According to one study"*: Shameek Rakshit et al., "The Burden of Medical Debt in the United States," Peterson-KFF Health System Tracker, February 12, 2024, https://www.healthsystemtracker.org/brief/the-burden-of-medical-debt-in-the-united-states/.

4 — WORK

83 *Roughly one-third of Americans rent*: U.S. Census Bureau, "Nearly Half of Renter Households Are Cost-Burdened, Proportions Differ by Race," September 12, 2024, https://www.census.gov/newsroom/press-releases/2024/renter-households-cost-burdened-race.html.

83 *Since 2019, rents have increased*: Anna Helhoski, "Rent Growth Outstrips Wages in Most U.S. Metros, New Report Shows," NerdWallet, May 8, 2024, https://www.nerdwallet.com/article/finance/rent-vs-income.

83 *one research project estimates*: Jerry Anthony, "Housing Affordability and Economic Growth," *Housing Policy Debate* 32, no. 3 (2022):

456–74, https://nlihc.org/sites/default/files/Housing_Affordability_Economic_Growth.pdf.

83 *Elevated housing costs*: Lauren A. Taylor, "Housing and Health: An Overview of the Literature," *Health Affairs Health Policy Brief*, June 7, 2018, https://www.healthaffairs.org/content/briefs/housing-and-health-overview-literature.

83 *770,000 Americans experience homelessness*: Claire Thornton, "How Many People Were Homeless in the US in 2024?," *USA Today*, December 27, 2024, https://www.usatoday.com/story/news/nation/2024/12/27/how-many-people-are-homeless-us-2024/77020773007/.

83 *communities where the median*: National Low Income Housing Coalition, "Zillow Research Examines Relationship Between Rent Affordability and Homelessness," NLIHC, December 11, 2018, https://nlihc.org/resource/zillow-research-examines-relationship-between-rent-affordability-and-homelessness.

97 *Seventy percent of Americans admit*: "Imposter Syndrome," *Psychology Today*, accessed April 21, 2025, https://www.psychologytoday.com/us/basics/imposter-syndrome.

101 *Sir James Dyson made 5,126 prototypes*: James Dyson, *Against the Odds: An Autobiography* (London: Texere Publishing, 2002).

101 *Jack Ma was rejected*: Jack Ma, interview by World Economic Forum, Davos, 2015, https://www.weforum.org/videos/alibaba-founder-jack-ma-harvard-rejected-me-10-times/.

103 *The New York Times even described*: Gary Rivlin, "A Founder at RedEnvelope Tries to Take Back Control," *New York Times*, August 2, 2004, https://www.nytimes.com/2004/08/02/business/a-founder-at-redenvelope-tries-to-take-back-control.html.

105 *Most hugely successful entrepreneurs*: Tim Chae, "Was Your First Startup a Small Outcome? Your Next Startup Is Much More Likely to Become a Unicorn," *Marker* (Medium), March 3, 2020, https://marker.medium.com/was-your-first-startup-a-small-Outcome-your-next-startup-is-much-more-likely-to-become-a-unicorn-28c438760f47.

105 *One study asked participants*: The Decision Lab, "The Sunk Cost Fallacy," accessed May 2025, https://thedecisionlab.com/biases/the-sunk-cost-fallacy.

106 *When Liverpool FC manager*: Liverpool FC, "Jürgen Klopp Announces Decision to Step Down as Liverpool Manager at End of Season," January 26, 2024, https://www.liverpoolfc.com/news/jurgen-klopp-announces-decision-step-down-liverpool-manager-end-season.

107 *"We are mites on a plum"*: Carl Sagan, interview by Steve Paikin, *The Agenda*, TVO, January 30, 1995, https://www.tvo.org/transcript/005584/interview-carl-sagan.
109 *more than four hundred nightclubs*: BBC News, "Calls to Save the UK's Ailing Nightclub Industry After Another Year of Closures," December 27, 2024, https://www.bbc.com/news/articles/czed9321l37o.
110 *Fewer than half feel a sense of community*: Elise A. Spenner and Tanya J. Vidhun, "Young Americans Oppose Trump, Report Economic Hardship in New IOP Poll," *Harvard Crimson*, April 23, 2025, https://www.thecrimson.com/article/2025/4/23/iop-poll-trump-policies/.

5 – HEALTH

115 *Nearly 60 percent of American*: Phil Edwards, "A Brief History of the Bizarre and Sadistic Presidential Fitness Test," Vox, April 24, 2015, https://www.vox.com/2015/4/24/8489501/presidential-fitness-test.
115 *obesity was correlated*: Centers for Disease Control and Prevention, "Obesity and COVID-19," accessed April 21, 2025, https://www.cdc.gov/obesity/data/obesity-and-covid-19.html.
116 *Obesity is heritable*: "Why People Become Overweight," Harvard Health Publishing, accessed April 21, 2025, https://www.health.harvard.edu/staying-healthy/why-people-become-overweight.
116 *$173 billion*: Centers for Disease Control and Prevention, "Adult Obesity Facts," last reviewed May 17, 2023, https://www.cdc.gov/obesity/adult-obesity-facts/index.html.
116 *Plus-size clothing*: Grand View Research, "Plus-Size Clothing Market Size, Share & Trends," accessed April 21, 2025, https://www.grandviewresearch.com/industry-analysis/plus-size-clothing-market-report.
116 *Japan, which has*: Aryn Baker, "Why Japan Has Such a Low Rate of Obesity," *Time*, February 29, 2024, https://time.com/6974579/japan-food-culture-low-obesity/.
116 *Strict rules govern*: Baker, "Why Japan Has Such a Low Rate."
116 *American armed service enrollment*: WAVY, "U.S. Military Sees Record-Breaking Low Recruitment Numbers," accessed April 21, 2025, https://www.wavy.com/news/military/u-s-military-sees-record-breaking-low-recruitment-numbers/.
117 *Around 77 percent require*: Thomas Novelly, "Even More Young Americans Are Unfit to Serve, a New Study Finds. Here's Why," Military.com, September 28, 2022, https://www.military.com/daily-news/2022/09

/28/new-pentagon-study-shows-77-of-young-americans-are-ineligible-military-service.html.

117 *The bad news is*: Jon Solomon, "Participation Trends," *State of Play 2024*, Aspen Institute's Project Play, October 2024, https://projectplay.org/state-of-play-2024-participation-trends.

117 *Among Black boys*: Solomon, "Participation Trends."

118 *"acceptable at a dance"*: Richard Reeves, "How Men Can Be Invaluable at the Dance," *Of Boys and Men* (Substack), accessed April 21, 2025, https://ofboysandmen.substack.com/p/how-men-can-be-invaluable-at-the.

118 *many exercise four to five times*: Lisa Eadicicco, *Business Insider*, "What 12 Top Tech Executives Do to Stay in Shape," *Inc.*, accessed April 21, 2025, https://www.inc.com/business-insider/what-12-top-tech-executives-do-to-stay-in-shape.html.

119 *weight control, increased energy*: Mayo Clinic Staff, "Exercise: 7 Benefits of Regular Physical Activity," Mayo Clinic, accessed April 21, 2025, https://www.mayoclinic.org/healthy-lifestyle/fitness/in-depth/exercise/art-20048389.

123 *Not an anomaly here*: "Exercising to Relax," Harvard Health Publishing, accessed April 21, 2025, https://www.health.harvard.edu/staying-healthy/exercising-to-relax.

123 *Exercise can even help*: "How We Can Exercise Away Addiction and Depression," *Psychology Today*, May 2024, https://www.psychologytoday.com/us/blog/addiction-outlook/202405/how-we-can-exercise-away-addiction-and-depression.

123 *Any exercise works*: "Exercising to Relax."

123 *a 2024 study shows*: Michael Noetel et al., "Effect of Exercise for Depression: Systematic Review and Network Meta-Analysis of Randomised Controlled Trials," *British Medical Journal* 384 (2024): e075847, https://www.bmj.com/content/384/bmj-2023-075847.

126 *Stepping outside*: Cassidy Randall, "Why Going Outside Is Good for Your Health, Especially Right Now," *Forbes*, April 9, 2020, https://www.forbes.com/sites/cassidyrandall/2020/04/09/why-going-outside-is-good-for-your-health-especially-right-now/.

126 *Exposure to sunlight*: Roma Parikh et al., "Skin Exposure to UVB Light Induces a Skin-Brain-Gonad Axis and Sexual Behavior," *Cell Reports* 36, no. 8 (2021): 109579, https://www.cell.com/cell-reports/fulltext/S2211-1247(21)01013-5.

127 *Spending two hours a week outside*: Mathew P. White et al., "Spending at Least 120 Minutes a Week in Nature Is Associated with Good Health

and Wellbeing," *Scientific Reports* 9, no. 7730 (2019), https://www.nature.com/articles/s41598-019-44097-3.

127 *Some doctors prescribe*: Perri Klass, "Writing Prescriptions to Play Outdoors," *New York Times*, July 16, 2018, https://www.nytimes.com/2018/07/16/well/writing-prescriptions-to-play-outdoors.html.

127 *The Swedes have a word*: BBC Worklife, "Friluftsliv: The Nordic Concept of Getting Outdoors," December 11, 2017, https://www.bbc.com/worklife/article/20171211-friluftsliv-the-nordic-concept-of-getting-outdoors.

133 *as Dorothy Parker said once*: Dorothy Parker, quoted in John Dugdale, "The Wicked Wit and Enigma of Dorothy Parker, 50 Years On," *Guardian*, June 16, 2017, https://www.theguardian.com/books/booksblog/2017/jun/16/the-wicked-wit-and-enigma-of-dorothy-parker-50-years-on.

138 *There are studies that high-potency*: National Academies of Sciences, Engineering, and Medicine, *The Health Effects of Cannabis and Cannabinoids: The Current State of Evidence and Recommendations for Research* (Washington, DC: The National Academies Press, 2017), https://www.ncbi.nlm.nih.gov/books/NBK425748/.

138 *Low amounts of THC*: Rhitu Chatterjee, "Highly Potent Weed Has Swept the Market, Raising Concerns About Health Risks," NPR, May 15, 2019, https://www.npr.org/sections/health-shots/2019/05/15/723656629/highly-potent-weed-has-swept-the-market-raising-concerns-about-health-risks.

138 *Adolescents are especially susceptible*: Chatterjee, "Highly Potent Weed."

138 *THC accompanied by high levels*: Evan A. Winiger et al., "Cannabis Use and Sleep: Expectations, Outcomes, and the Role of Age," *Addictive Behaviors* 112 (2021): 106642, https://www.ncbi.nlm.nih.gov/pmc/articles/PMC7572650/.

140 *Men are more likely*: National Institute on Drug Abuse, "Sex Differences in Substance Use," Research Report Series, https://nida.nih.gov/publications/research-reports/substance-use-in-women/sex-differences-in-substance-use.

140 *They're more prone than women*: Centers for Disease Control and Prevention, "Alcohol Use Effects on Men's and Women's Health," CDC, January 31, 2025, https://www.cdc.gov/alcohol/about-alcohol-use/alcohol-and-sex-considerations.html.

140 *Two-thirds of all opioid-related*: National Institute on Drug Abuse, "Overdose Death Rates," NIDA, January 2024, https://nida.nih.gov/research-topics/trends-statistics/overdose-death-rates#Fig1.

140 *Twenty million Americans struggle*: Anders Bergman, "207 Gambling Addiction Statistics & Facts 2025," QuitGamble.com, March 28, 2025, https://quitgamble.com/gambling-addiction-statistics-and-facts/.

140 *Gambling addiction in men*: Haroon Siddique, "Problem Gamblers at 15 Times Higher Risk of Suicide, Study Finds," *Guardian*, March 13, 2019, https://www.theguardian.com/society/2019/mar/13/problem-gamblers-at-15-times-higher-risk-of-suicide-study-finds.

140 *Sports gambling is now legal*: Cassie Bottorff, "Americans Are Losing Big on Sports Betting," Investopedia, April 2, 2024, https://www.investopedia.com/americans-sports-betting-losing-8768618.

140 *In 2024, 72 percent*: Statista Research Department, "Share of Sports Betting Participants in the United States in 2024, by Gender," Statista, April 2024, https://www.statista.com/statistics/1105283/sport-gambling-interest-gender/.

141 *As my NYU colleague*: Christine Rosen, "'The Anxious Generation' Review: Apps, Angst and Adolescence," *Wall Street Journal*, March 22, 2024, https://www.wsj.com/arts-culture/books/the-anxious-generation-review-apps-angst-and-adolescence-be910482.

141 *So far, the results are*: Jean M. Twenge, "Increases in Depression, Self-Harm, and Suicide Among U.S. Adolescents After 2012 and Links to Technology Use: Possible Mechanisms," *Psychological Inquiry* 33, no. 3 (2022): 181–94, https://pmc.ncbi.nlm.nih.gov/articles/PMC9169592/.

141 *The suicide rate among teens*: Jonathan Haidt, introduction to "Suicide Rates Are Now Higher Among Young People Than the Middle-Aged," by Jean M. Twenge, *After Babel* (newsletter), February 5, 2024, https://www.afterbabel.com/p/suicide-rates-are-now-higher-among.

141 *Teens who are on social media*: U.S. Department of Health and Human Services, *Social Media and Youth Mental Health: The U.S. Surgeon General's Advisory*, 2023, https://www.hhs.gov/surgeongeneral/reports-and-publications/youth-mental-health/social-media/index.html.

141 *Is it any wonder Tim Cook*: Olivia Solon, "Tim Cook: I Don't Want My Nephew on a Social Network," *Guardian*, January 19, 2018, https://www.theguardian.com/technology/2018/jan/19/tim-cook-i-dont-want-my-nephew-on-a-social-network.

141 *And about one in ten*: D. A. Gentile, "Pathological Video-Game Use Among Youth Ages 8 to 18: A National Study," *Psychological Science* 20, no. 6 (2009): 594–602, https://pubmed.ncbi.nlm.nih.gov/19476590/.

141 *And about one in ten*: Natalia Suárez-Álvarez et al., "Video Game Addiction and Depression: A Systematic Review and Meta-Analysis,"

International Journal of Environmental Research and Public Health 20, no. 6 (2023): 4765, https://www.ncbi.nlm.nih.gov/pmc/articles/PMC10065366/.

141 *50 percent of all teenagers*: Yitz Diena, "75 Cell Phone Addiction: Facts & Statistics," Ambitions ABA, accessed May 2025, https://www.ambitionsaba.com/resources/cell-phone-addiction-facts-statistics.

141 *Fast food also triggers*: Cheryl D. Fryar et al., "Fast Food Intake Among Children and Adolescents in the United States, 2015–2018," *NCHS Data Brief* no. 375 (August 2020): 1–8, https://www.cdc.gov/nchs/data/databriefs/db375-h.pdf.

142 *At least twenty-five states*: Arianna Prothero et al., "Which States Ban or Restrict Cellphones in Schools?," *Education Week*, June 25, 2024, https://www.edweek.org/technology/which-states-ban-or-restrict-cellphones-in-schools/2024/06.

142 *roughly three-quarters of schools*: Lauraine Langreo, "Cellphone Bans Can Ease Students' Stress and Anxiety, Educators Say," *Education Week*, October 24, 2023, https://www.edweek.org/leadership/cellphone-bans-can-ease-students-stress-and-anxiety-educators-say/2023/10.

142 *Yondr, a firm that makes*: Andrew R. Chow, "Cell Phone Pouches Promise to Improve Focus at School. Kids Aren't Convinced," *Time*, March 27, 2024, https://time.com/6959626/yondr-schools-cell-phones/.

142 *An "electronics fast"*: Victoria L. Dunckley, "Screentime Is Making Kids Moody, Crazy, and Lazy," *Psychology Today*, August 27, 2015, https://www.psychologytoday.com/us/blog/mental-wealth/201508/screentime-is-making-kids-moody-crazy-and-lazy.

142 *Lowering your dopamine threshold*: WebMD Editorial Contributors, "What Is Dopamine?," WebMD, accessed May 2025, https://www.webmd.com/mental-health/what-is-dopamine#1.

143 *Since 2017, Congress has held*: Kaitlyn Tiffany, "Protecting Children Online Is Nearly Impossible," *Atlantic*, October 12, 2023, https://www.theatlantic.com/technology/archive/2023/10/protect-children-online-social-media-internet/675825/.

143 *Senator Dick Durbin had it right*: U.S. Senate Judiciary Committee, "Durbin Delivers Opening Statement During Senate Judiciary Committee Hearing Examining Big Tech's Failures to Protect Kids from Sexual Exploitation Online," January 31, 2024, https://www.judiciary.senate.gov/press/releases/durbin-delivers-opening-statement-during-senate-judiciary-committee-hearing-examining-big-techs-failures-to-protect-kids-from-sexual-exploitation-online.

143 *Men today have a higher mortality rate*: Leana S. Wen, "We're Missing a Huge Piece of the Health Gender Gap," *Washington Post*, August 27, 2024, https://www.washingtonpost.com/opinions/2024/08/27/men-health-crisis-gender-gaps/.

143 *Boys and men are four times*: William Kremer, "Why More Men Kill Themselves Than Women," *BBC Future*, March 13, 2019, https://www.bbc.com/future/article/20190313-why-more-men-kill-themselves-than-women.

6 – FRIENDSHIP

150 *Despite its health benefits*: Daniel A. Cox, *The State of American Friendship: Change, Challenges, and Loss*, Survey Center on American Life, May 2021, https://www.americansurveycenter.org/research/the-state-of-american-friendship-change-challenges-and-loss/.

150 *Since 1990, the percentage*: Cox, *State of American Friendship*.

151 *Young adults' loneliness rates*: U.S. Department of Health and Human Services, *Our Epidemic of Loneliness and Isolation: The U.S. Surgeon General's Advisory on the Healing Effects of Social Connection and Community*, 2023, https://www.hhs.gov/sites/default/files/surgeon-general-social-connection-advisory.pdf.

151 *In the past decade, teen depression*: Sylia Wilson and Nathalie M. Dumornay, "Rising Rates of Adolescent Depression in the United States: Challenges and Opportunities in the 2020s," *Journal of Adolescent Health* 70, no. 3 (March 2022): 354–55, https://www.ncbi.nlm.nih.gov/pmc/articles/PMC8868033/.

151 *It's worse for men*: Daniel A. Cox, "American Men Suffer a Friendship Recession," *Survey Center on American Life*, July 6, 2021, https://www.americansurveycenter.org/commentary/american-men-suffer-a-friendship-recession/.

151 *a trend that predates Covid*: American Psychological Association, "COVID-19 Pandemic Led to Increase in Loneliness Around the World," May 2022, https://www.apa.org/news/press/releases/2022/05/covid-19-increase-loneliness.

151 *In a 2021 survey*: Catherine Pearson, "Why Is It So Hard for Men to Make Close Friends?," *New York Times*, November 28, 2022, https://www.nytimes.com/2022/11/28/well/family/male-friendship-loneliness.html.

151 *That same survey found*: Pearson, "Why Is It So Hard?"

151 *A 2023 study*: Equimundo, *State of American Men 2023: From Crisis and Confusion to Hope*, https://www.equimundo.org/resources/state-of-american-men/.

Notes

151 *Among couples in heterosexual*: Kasley Killam, "The Hidden Costs of Men's Social Isolation," *Scientific American*, July 2022, https://www.scientificamerican.com/article/the-hidden-costs-of-mens-social-isolation/.

151 *When a relationship ends*: Killam, "Hidden Costs."

152 *According to one 2022 study*: Catherine Pearson, "Text Your Friends. It Matters More Than You Think," *New York Times*, July 11, 2022, https://www.nytimes.com/2022/07/11/well/family/check-in-text-friendship.html.

153 *The economist Raj Chetty*: Raj Chetty et al., "Social Capital II: Determinants of Economic Connectedness," Opportunity Insights, July 2022, https://opportunityinsights.org/wp-content/uploads/2022/07/socialcapital_nontech.pdf.

153 *Unemployed people who volunteer*: Christopher Spera et al., "Volunteering as a Pathway to Employment: Does Volunteering Increase Odds of Finding a Job for the Out of Work?," Corporation for National and Community Service (2013), https://www.americorps.gov/sites/default/files/evidence_exchange/FR_2013_VolunteeringasaPathwaytoEmployment_1.pdf.

153 *aided by the "social capital"*: Christopher Spera et al., "Volunteering as a Pathway to Employment: Does Volunteering Increase Odds of Finding a Job for the out of Work?," Corporation for National and Community Service, June 2013, https://americorps.gov/sites/default/files/evidenceexchange/FR_2013_VolunteeringasaPathwaytoEmployment_1.pdf.

153 *Regions with greater civic engagement*: National Conference on Citizenship, *Civic Health and Unemployment: The Case Builds*, 2011, https://ncoc.org/wp-content/uploads/2015/04/2011UnemploymentCHI.pdf.

153 *communities to which the residents*: Knight Foundation, "Got Love for Your Community? It May Create Economic Growth, Gallup Study Says," November 15, 2010, https://knightfoundation.org/press/releases/got-love-for-your-community-it-may-create-economic/.

153 *The CDC estimates*: New York State Office for the Aging, "Combating Social Isolation and Loneliness," https://aging.ny.gov/combating-social-isolation#.

155 *Single men could die*: University of Louisville study, as reported in Rosemary Brennan, "This Just In: Do Singles Have a Higher 'Risk of Death' Than Their Married Counterparts?!," *Glamour*, August 2011, https://www.glamour.com/story/this-just-in-do-singles-have-a.

155 *Mortality risk is 20 percent*: Julianne Holt-Lunstad et al., "Loneliness and Social Isolation as Risk Factors for Mortality: A Meta-Analytic

Review," *Perspectives on Psychological Science* 10, no. 2 (2015): 227–37, https://journals.sagepub.com/doi/10.1177/1745691614568352.

155 *and 32 percent higher for people who live alone*: Holt-Lunstad et al., "Loneliness and Social Isolation."

155 *Basically, men with fewer friends*: Kayla Mansour et al., "Social Network Investment of Men: Cross-Sectional and Longitudinal Associations with Mental Health Problems," *Applied Psychology: Health and Well-Being* 16, no. 1 (February 2024): 138–57, https://iaap-journals.onlinelibrary.wiley.com/doi/full/10.1111/aphw.12475.

158 *Kipling probably said it best*: Rudyard Kipling, "If—," Poetry Foundation, https://www.poetryfoundation.org/poems/46473/if---.

168 *Archaeologists recently discovered*: Brigit Katz, "Traces of 13,000-Year-Old Beer Found in Israel," *Smithsonian*, September 13, 2018, https://www.smithsonianmag.com/smart-news/traces-13000-year-old-beer-found-israel-180970282/.

168 *there is archaeological evidence*: David Kindy, "Beer Flowed Freely at Gatherings in the Jordan Valley 7,000 Years Ago," *Smithsonian*, January 5, 2022, https://www.smithsonianmag.com/smart-news/beer-flowed-freely-at-gatherings-in-jordan-valley-7000-years-ago-180979323/.

168 *Everyone but the liquor*: Centers for Disease Control and Prevention, "Facts About U.S. Deaths from Excessive Alcohol Use," August 6, 2024, https://www.cdc.gov/alcohol/facts-stats/index.html.

169 *the number one risk factor*: National Institute on Alcohol Abuse and Alcoholism, "Global Burden," https://www.niaaa.nih.gov/alcohols-effects-health/alcohol-topics/alcohol-facts-and-statistics/global-burden.

169 *Thirty million Americans*: The Pew Charitable Trusts, "America's Most Common Drug Problem? Unhealthy Alcohol Use," December 2024, https://www.pewtrusts.org/en/research-and-analysis/fact-sheets/2024/12/americas-most-common-drug-problem-unhealthy-alcohol-use.

169 *in addition to killing*: National Institute on Alcohol Abuse and Alcoholism, "Alcohol-Related Emergencies and Deaths in the United States," https://www.niaaa.nih.gov/alcohols-effects-health/alcohol-topics-z/alcohol-facts-and-statistics/alcohol-related-emergencies-and-deaths-united-states.

169 *alcohol leads to*: The Pew Charitable Trusts, "America's Most Common Drug Problem?"

169 *Even light drinking can increase*: World Health Organization, "No Level of Alcohol Consumption Is Safe for Our Health," January 4, 2023, https://www.who.int/europe/news/item/04-01-2023-no-level-of-alcohol-consumption-is-safe-for-our-health.

7 – SEX, LOVE, MARRIAGE

180 *I once saw a study*: Stephanie Pappas, John-Tyler Binfet et al., "High School Students' Conceptualizations of Kindness: A Mixed-Methods Portrait," *Social and Emotional Learning: Research, Practice, and Policy* (2025), https://doi.org/10.1016/j.sel.2025.100089.

184 *Once married, one's household*: Elizabeth Matsangou, "For Richer, for Poorer: The Economics of Marriage," World Finance, https://www.worldfinance.com/wealth-management/for-richer-for-poorer-the-economics-of-marriage.

184 *Married couples, by their fifties*: W. Bradford Wilcox, "Two Is Wealthier Than One: Marital Status and Wealth Outcomes Among Preretirement Adults," Institute for Family Studies, December 1, 2021, https://ifstudies.org/blog/two-is-wealthier-than-one-marital-status-and-wealth-outcomes-among-preretirement-adults-.

184 *Married people live longer*: Robert H. Shmerling, "The Health Advantages of Marriage," Harvard Health Publishing, November 30, 2016, https://www.health.harvard.edu/blog/the-health-advantages-of-marriage-2016113010667.

184 *and are happier*: Shawn Grover and John F. Helliwell, "How's Life at Home? New Evidence on Marriage and the Set Point for Happiness," *Journal of Happiness Studies* 20 (2019): 373–90, https://link.springer.com/article/10.1007/s10902-017-9941-3.

184 *Higher marriage rates*: Aparna Mathur, "The Family Foundations of Economic Growth," *Forbes*, October 30, 2015, https://www.forbes.com/sites/aparnamathur/2015/10/30/the-family-foundations-of-economic-growth/.

184 *and a reduction in child poverty*: Robert Rector, "Marriage: America's Greatest Weapon Against Child Poverty," The Heritage Foundation, September 5, 2012, https://www.heritage.org/poverty-and-inequality/report/marriage-americas-greatest-weapon-against-child-poverty.

185 *In 1980, the figure was*: Lydia Saad, "Americans' Preference for Larger Families Highest Since 1971," Gallup, July 31, 2023, https://news.gallup.com/poll/511238/americans-preference-larger-families-highest-1971.aspx.

186 *On Hinge, the top 10 percent*: Dan Kopf, "These Statistics Show Why It's So Hard to Be an Average Man on Dating Apps," Quartz, August 15, 2017, https://qz.com/1051462/these-statistics-show-why-its-so-hard-to-be-an-average-man-on-dating-apps.

186 *The bottom 80 percent*: Worst-Online-Dater, "Tinder Experiments II: Guys, Unless You Are Really Hot You Are Probably Better Off Not Wasting Your Time on Tinder—A Quantitative Socio-Economic Study," Medium, March 25, 2015, https://medium.com/@worstonlinedater/tinder-experiments-ii-guys-unless-you-are-really-hot-you-are-probably-better-off-not-wasting-your-2ddf370a6e9a.

186 *Only 34 percent*: Risa Gelles-Watnick, "For Valentine's Day, 5 Facts About Single Americans," Pew Research Center, February 8, 2023, https://www.pewresearch.org/short-reads/2023/02/08/for-valentines-day-5-facts-about-single-americans/.

186 *The reasons include*: Rachel Wolfe, "American Women Are Giving Up on Marriage," *Wall Street Journal*, March 21, 2025, https://www.wsj.com/lifestyle/relationships/american-women-are-giving-up-on-marriage-54840971.

187 *Between 1970 and 2011*: Michael Greenstone and Adam Looney, "The Marriage Gap: The Impact of Economic and Technological Change on Marriage Rates," The Hamilton Project (2012), https://www.hamiltonproject.org/publication/post/the-marriage-gap-the-impact-of-economic-and-technological-change-on-marriage-rates/.

187 *In the past forty years*: Daniel A. Cox, *Emerging Trends and Enduring Patterns in American Family Life*, Survey Center on American Life, February 2021, https://www.americansurveycenter.org/research/emerging-trends-and-enduring-patterns-in-american-family-life/.

187 *College-educated men*: Social Security Administration data, as cited on PolitiFact, March 8, 2023, https://www.politifact.com/factchecks/2023/mar/08/stanley-litow/strong-support-for-notion-that-a-bachelors-degree/.

187 *A college degree also increases*: Kim Parker and Renee Stapler, "As U.S. Marriage Rate Hovers at 50%, Education Gap in Marital Status Widens," Pew Research Center, September 14, 2017, https://www.pewresearch.org/short-reads/2017/09/14/as-u-s-marriage-rate-hovers-at-50-education-gap-in-marital-status-widens/.

187 *There are now just 2.1*: Central Intelligence Agency, "Dependency Ratios," *The World Factbook*, accessed May 2025, https://www.cia.gov/the-world-factbook/field/dependency-ratios/.

188 *While violent crime*: John Grimlach, "What the Data Says About Crime in the U.S.," Pew Research Center, April 24, 2024, https://www.pewresearch.org/short-reads/2024/04/24/what-the-data-says-about-crime-in-the-us.

188 *men are already more prone*: David Barczak, "Conspiracy and Gender," University of Delaware Research Office, July 26, 2020, https://research.udel.edu/2020/07/26/conspiracy-and-gender/.

192 *Some estimates put porn-related*: Sebastian Anthony, "Just How Big Are Porn Sites?," ExtremeTech, March 2, 2012, https://www.extremetech.com/internet/123929-just-how-big-are-porn-sites.

193 *The most recent figures*: Scott Galloway, "Porn," Medium, March 21, 2025, https://medium.com/@profgalloway/porn-6294dd8b5b8e.

193 *In a study of two thousand adults*: Joshua B. Grubbs, Samuel W. Kraus, and Samuel L. Perry, "Self-Reported Addiction to Pornography in a Nationally Representative Sample: The Roles of Use Habits, Religiousness, and Moral Incongruence," *Journal of Behavioral Addictions* 8, no. 1 (2019): 88–93, https://pmc.ncbi.nlm.nih.gov/articles/PMC7044607/.

193 *Meanwhile, OnlyFans generated*: Matthew Ball, "Breaking Down OnlyFans' Stunning Economics," MatthewBall.co, September 7, 2024, https://www.matthewball.co/all/fansprofitandloss.

193 *The firm has more than*: Mary Harrington, "Female Celebrities Are Making Millions on OnlyFans. Will They Regret It?," *Wall Street Journal*, https://www.wsj.com/lifestyle/female-celebrities-are-making-millions-on-onlyfans-will-they-regret-it-f35a560c.

193 *More research is needed*: Ana J. Bridges et al., "Pornography Use and Sexual Objectification of Others," *Violence Against Women* 30, no. 1 (January 2024): 228–48, https://doi.org/10.1177/10778012231207041.

193 *A longitudinal survey*: Jochen Peter and Patti M. Valkenburg, "Adolescents' Exposure to Sexually Explicit Internet Material and Notions of Women as Sex Objects: Assessing Causality and Underlying Processes," *Journal of Communication* 59, no. 3 (2009): 407–33, https://academic.oup.com/joc/article-abstract/59/3/407/4098518.

195 *According to Dr. Anna Lembke*: Anna Lembke, interview by Scott Galloway, *The Prof G Show*, YouTube video, 1:01:45, February 2025, https://www.youtube.com/watch?v=ZtXkfMw_uMI.

199 *Women initiate most divorces*: American Sociological Association, "Women More Likely Than Men to Initiate Divorces, but Not Non-Marital Breakups," August 22, 2015, https://www.asanet.org/women-more-likely-men-initiate-divorces-not-non-marital-breakups/.

199 *The data on long-term psychological*: Thomas Leopold, "Gender Differences in the Consequences of Divorce: A Study of Multiple Outcomes,"

Demography 55, no. 3 (2018): 769–97, https://pmc.ncbi.nlm.nih.gov/articles/PMC5992251/.

199 *Children of divorced parents*: Brian D'Onofrio and Robert Emery, "Parental Divorce or Separation and Children's Mental Health," *World Psychiatry* 18, no. 1 (2019): 100–101, https://pmc.ncbi.nlm.nih.gov/articles/PMC6313686/.

200 *They're also less likely*: D'Onofrio and Emery, "Parental Divorce or Separation."

200 *Relationships that breed*: Elizabeth Gershoff and Andrew Grogan-Kaylor, "Parental Divorce or Separation and Children's Mental Health," *Pediatrics & Child Health* 23, no. 2 (2018): e133–37, https://www.ncbi.nlm.nih.gov/pmc/articles/PMC6313686/.

202 *Studies show that forgiveness*: Scott R. Braithwaite et al., "Trait Forgiveness and Enduring Vulnerabilities: Neuroticism and Catastrophizing Influence Relationship Satisfaction via Less Forgiveness," *Personality and Individual Differences* 94 (2016): 237–46, https://fincham.info/papers/2016-paid.pdf.

202 *Caregivers are the most important*: David L. Roth et al., "Reduced Mortality Rates Among Caregivers: Does Family Caregiving Provide a Stress-Buffering Effect?," *Psychology and Aging* 33, no. 4 (2018): 619–29, https://pmc.ncbi.nlm.nih.gov/articles/PMC6002922/.

202 *the so-called Four Horsemen*: The Gottman Institute, "Marriage and Couples—Research," https://www.gottman.com/about/research/couples/.

203 *Ditto for emotional withdrawal*: Gottman Institute, "Marriage and Couples—Research."

203 *Note: 85 percent of all stonewallers*: Gottman Institute, "Marriage and Couples—Research."

8 — FATHERHOOD

206 *New dads' testosterone*: Darby E. Saxbe et al., "Prenatal Testosterone Synchrony in First-Time Parents Predicts Fathers' Testosterone Decline and Postpartum Relationship Investment," *Hormones and Behavior* 154 (2023): 105342, https://www.sciencedirect.com/science/article/abs/pii/S0018506X23001381.

206 *Their balls shrink, too*: Stephanie Pappas, "Smaller Testicles Linked to Better Fathers," *Scientific American*, September 10, 2013, https://www.scientificamerican.com/article/smaller-testicles-linked-fathers/.

208 *In a 2017 piece published on Medium*: Mark Greene, "The Lack of Gentle Platonic Touch in Men's Lives Is a Killer," Medium, May 28, 2018, https://remakingmanhood.medium.com/the-lack-of-gentle-platonic-touch-in-mens-lives-is-a-killer-5cc8eb144001.

221 *Our brain stands at attention*: David Eagleman, "Brain Time," Eagleman.com, https://eagleman.com/latest/brain-time/.

227 *Today, women are the primary breadwinners*: Sarah Jane Glynn, "Breadwinning Mothers Continue to Be the U.S. Norm," Center for American Progress, May 10, 2019, https://www.americanprogress.org/article/breadwinning-mothers-continue-u-s-norm/.

227 *the percentage of women*: Richard Fry et al., "In a Growing Share of U.S. Marriages, Husbands and Wives Earn About the Same," Pew Research Center, April 13, 2023, https://www.pewresearch.org/social-trends/2023/04/13/in-a-growing-share-of-u-s-marriages-husbands-and-wives-earn-about-the-same/.

227 *Among married-couple families*: U.S. Bureau of Labor Statistics, "Employment Characteristics of Families—2023," April 18, 2024, https://www.bls.gov/news.release/pdf/famee.pdf.

230 *Dads, I might add*: The Law Office of Nicholas W. Richardson, "Fathers and Mothers: Child Custody Myths," Dads Divorce Law, https://www.dadsdivorcelaw.com/blog/fathers-and-mothers-child-custody-myths.

234 *Boys especially have*: Daniel A. Abrams et al., "A Neurodevelopmental Shift in Reward Circuitry from Mother's to Nonfamilial Voices in Adolescence," *Journal of Neuroscience* 14, no. 20, May 18, 2022, https://www.jneurosci.org/content/42/20/4164.

10 – LIFE IS SO RICH

250 *A study shows that one in ten*: Dara N. Greenwood, "Fame, Facebook, and Twitter: How Attitudes About Fame Predict Frequency and Nature of Social Media Use," *Psychology of Popular Media Culture* 2, no. 4 (2013): 222–36, https://doi.org/10.1037/ppm0000013.

257 *Crying may have an evolutionary purpose*: Alix Spiegel, "Teary-Eyed Evolution: Crying Serves a Purpose," NPR, August 23, 2010, https://www.npr.org/2010/08/23/129329054/teary-eyed-evolution-crying-serves-a-purpose.

257 *One way to solve this*: BabyCenter Editors, "Harvey Karp's Happiest Baby Method for Baby Sleep and Soothing," BabyCenter, January 17,

2024, https://www.babycenter.com/baby/sleep/harvey-karps-happiest-baby-method-for-baby-sleep-and-soothin_10373838#articlesection1.

257 *Swaddle, Side-stomach position*: Harvey Karp, "The Science Behind the 5 S's," Happiest Baby, https://www.happiestbaby.com/blogs/baby/science-5-s-s.

About the Author

SCOTT GALLOWAY is a professor of marketing at NYU's Stern School of Business and a serial entrepreneur. He was named one of the world's best business professors by *Poets&Quants*. Scott has founded nine companies, including Prophet, RedEnvelope, L2, and Section, where he also teaches. He is the *New York Times* bestselling author of *The Four*, *The Algebra of Happiness*, *Post Corona*, *Adrift*, and *The Algebra of Wealth*. Scott has served on the boards of directors of the New York Times Company, Urban Outfitters, Berkeley's Haas School of Business, Panera Bread, and Ledger. He has won multiple Webby and best podcast awards, and his books have been translated into twenty-eight languages. Across his *Prof G Pod*, *Prof G Markets*, and *Pivot* podcasts, his *No Mercy/No Malice* newsletter, and his YouTube channel, Scott reaches millions.